Strategic Marketing

How To Achieve Independence And Prosperity In Your Mental Health Practice

Kalman M. Heller, PhD

> **Running a successful solo or
> small group practice
> when everyone says
> it can't be done anymore.**

Professional Resource Press
Sarasota, Florida

Published by Professional Resource Press
(An imprint of Professional Resource Exchange, Inc.)
Post Office Box 15560
Sarasota, FL 34277-1560

The copy editor for this book was Patricia Rockwood, the managing editor was Debra Fink, the production coordinator was Laurie Girsch, and the cover was created by Jami S. Stinnet.

Library of Congress Cataloging-in-Publication Data

Heller, Kalman M.
    Strategic marketing : how to achieve independence and prosperity in your mental health practice / Kalman M. Heller
        p.   cm.
    "Running a successful solo or small group practice when everyone says it can't be done anymore."
    Includes bibliographical references (p.).
    ISBN 1-56887-031-0 (alk. paper)
    1. Psychotherapy--Marketing. 2. Mental health services--Marketing. I. Title.
RC465.5.H45 1997
616.89'0068--dc21   97-25932
                                            CIP

Dedication

To My Mother

Preface

This book approaches the issue of generating a successful private practice solely through a marketing model. It conveys an optimistic outlook that has become all too rare in today's managed-care-dominated marketplace. The book makes three promises. If you develop a marketing-driven practice, you will (a) become a more competent therapist, (b) increase your referrals and revenues, and (c) have more fun. How can I make these promises? Easy. I just described the last several years of my professional life!

I wish to thank Roberta Clarke and Ethan Pollack for their helpful feedback on my first draft. I also want to thank my secretary, Tracy Welch, who kept putting together the final versions of each draft. Most of all, a very special thanks to my wife, Ellen, for her input, encouragement, and support through the long process required in translating a dream into a published book.

Kalman M. Heller, PhD
Needham, Massachusetts

Table of Contents

Strategic Marketing

How To Achieve Independence And Prosperity In Your Mental Health Practice

Running a successful solo or
small group practice
when everyone says
it can't be done anymore.

1

The Challenge

"It was the best of times, it was the worst of times."
— Charles Dickens, *A Tale of Two Cities*

A new myth is being perpetrated on private practitioners across the land: *Big is beautiful. Big is necessary. The solo practice is dead. Long live vertically integrated systems and capitation.* This book is going to present a much more optimistic viewpoint. There is lots of business out there — enough for everyone, if you just know how to find it. This book will explain how you can do that.

Nick Cummings, one of the leading voices of the managed care industry, predicts that by the year 2000, 25% to 50% of PhD psychologists will be out of business ("A Look Ahead," 1996). Alan Savitz, medical director of Human Affairs International, also predicts that within 10 to 15 years, 50% of all mental health providers will be out of business ("Future Trends," 1993). This vision, shared by many other leaders in the managed care field, is commonly referred to as the industrialization of mental health care. In this model, a handful of companies dominate the field, and the survivors are those who

1

either are employed by these companies or have formed "supergroups" which contract with the managed care firms. The headline of a recent issue of *Managed Care Strategies* reads "Too Many Therapists and Not Enough Work" (1995, p.1). In the meantime, more than 20% of therapists in a recent poll ("Fee, Practice," 1995) said they were considering dropping out of the profession. Articles in nearly every professional newsletter contain complaints by therapists about reduced referrals or about doing more work for less pay. The field seems to be populated by many discouraged practitioners.

The responsibility for this changed climate does not lie solely with managed care companies. The percentage of corporate and government expenses devoted to health care has risen sharply over past decades, creating a demand for not merely controlling but also reducing these costs. There is debate, however, about the role of mental health costs in this problem. Monica Oss, among others, claims that behavioral health care costs have remained rather constant over the past 20 years, with treatment costs generally averaging between 9% and 11% of total health care costs (Sipkoff, 1995). Most of those costs are for inpatient care, meaning that outpatient psychotherapy services have generally accounted for about 2% to 3% of total health care costs. Many therapists feel that outpatient therapy is not the place to try to make major savings, citing (a) the nearly 50% prevalence rate of mental disorders for American adults (McBride, 1995), (b) the estimate that affective disorders alone cost industry nearly $24 billion in lost productivity (Yandrick & Oss, 1994), and (c) the fact that psychotherapy reduces medical expenditures by at least 20% (Sipkoff, 1995). With *Consumer Reports* ("Mental Health," 1995) joining a lengthening list of psychotherapy research reports claiming that psychotherapy really does help people, it is frustrating to see a system emerging that appears to be making it more difficult to obtain therapy. This is especially a concern because the same literature on the effectiveness of psychotherapy also reports that the majority of people (60% to 70%) who have a diagnosable mental health disorder are not seeking help from a mental health professional.

Despite all the financial, administrative, and ethical issues posed by managed care, its impact must not be viewed as entirely negative. As mental health professionals, we are being challenged to demonstrate greater accountability for the effectiveness of our work, to become more conscious of time and cost factors, and to become more creative in developing services that may better meet the needs of consumers. In other words, we are being asked to operate as service businesses. Where this book disagrees with all the current negativity pervading the industry is its vision that there is ample opportunity for solo and small group practices not merely to survive but to thrive. The key to achieving this success is to approach your practice as a small business, learn the basic concepts about how to market a small business, and then let your creative juices flow.

Many mental health professionals feel repulsed by the notion of being "in business," while others feel they are not suited to learn about marketing. I will address these concerns in more detail later; suffice it to say that when I have conducted workshops on this topic for practitioners like yourselves, the workshop invariably concludes with a room full of excited, optimistic converts ready to change their ways of thinking about and operating their practices. The feedback to date is that these changes result in achieving more success.

Several years ago I was beginning to feel the pinch of practicing in a geographic area that has one of the highest per capita ratios of therapists to the general population. The intense competition and the early glimmerings of managed care were just starting to be reflected in the first downward trend in number of referrals since I began my full-time practice in 1973. I made a decision to treat my practice as a service business and to teach myself about marketing. I am thankful to some early pioneers in this concept who gave me impetus and direction: Susan Sturdivant, James Schulman, and Monica Oss. The most important reason for you to read this book is that I know firsthand that what I am about to teach you does work.

In the past 5 years, compared to the previous 5 years, by applying the principles set forth in the remaining chapters, I have increased my referrals by 50%! This has happened despite the fact that the Greater Boston area has one of the highest market penetration rates by health maintenance organizations (HMOs) of any city in the country — and I do not belong to *any* of the four major players. Even more dramatic is the fact that in the past 3 years, my annual rate of referrals is double what my average annual rate had been during the first 19 years of my practice. And I have always been busy.

I do belong to a group. I do believe that a medium-sized group (10 to 15 therapists) is probably the most efficient and fun way to practice. But our group is organized around the principle of maintaining individual practices in the context of a professional association; to date, most of the success of my practice has not been based on my membership in the group. I strongly believe that if you want to operate the most traditional of all practices — going solo out of an office in your home — it can still be done.

This should be an exciting time in our field. The debates about managed care have forced our national organizations to become more political and educational. Never before have politicians or the public been so constantly bombarded with information about the value of mental health services. The response has generally been substantial support for mental health becoming a significant component of all future health care. The managed care horror stories are slowly but surely creating a public and, most importantly, private business backlash that inevitably will result in some degree of regulation, mandated or voluntary, that should eventually improve the context in which we will practice. In fact, there are literally hundreds of managed care regulatory bills that have been introduced this year at the state and federal levels.

We teach our patients that times of crisis become opportunities for change. Thus, we are also going to have to change the way we practice if we are to be successful. But the bottom line is that there are more ways to practice, more people who need and want our services, and new skills available to achieve success. This book simply makes it clear that you don't have to "sell out" to big business in order to maintain or create the small but successful practice that is your chosen way to help others. Being a therapist is one of the most challenging yet gratifying careers. It is a life dedicated to improving the quality of life for others. Don't let the uncertainties of these turbulent times stop you from your dedication to being a quality member of a helping profession.

2

Six Reasons to Learn Marketing Skills

1. The practice of psychotherapy involves delivering services for a fee. Delivering services for a fee is a business, just like any other service business. Regardless of whatever motivates you to be a therapist, patients are customers and you are a businessperson. Therefore, you need knowledge about how to run a business if you are likely to be successful.

2. Intense competition: Most metropolitan areas have high numbers of therapists from all disciplines. Licensing laws have been continually broadened to allow more therapists to be eligible for third-party payments, and many of those will accept lower fees than established therapists. Meanwhile, managed care affects more than 50% of all health services and brings with it restrictive panels, reduced fees, and an increasing influence over clinical decisions. Very soon, all health care services are likely to be managed to some degree. HMOs, which represent the most intrusive form of managed care, already have over 50 million members (more than 25% of all insured employees) and continue

to grow at a rapid pace. All these forces are serious threats to your ability to maintain or grow your practice.

3. On the positive side, there is a huge mental health marketplace that is still largely underdeveloped. Outpatient psychotherapy and related services are a $10 billion industry. This means that in order to gross $100,000, you need only a 0.000001% market share! More important, it is estimated that at any given moment, 20% to 30% of the population has a diagnosable mental health disorder, but only about 25% to 35% of those people seek help from a mental health practitioner. The majority either do nothing or talk to their physicians (which, unfortunately, may be worse than doing nothing), their clergy, or their friends. As a profession, we have done a very poor job of educating the majority of the people about what we do and how it can help them. This is changing, however; there has been a steady and significant annual increase in the percentage of the population seeking mental health services. Marketing skills will enable you to better inform others of the benefits of your services and to reach deeper into the untapped portions of the marketplace, not only as therapists but in a wider range of income-generating roles. And bear in mind that 20% of patients pay cash, with some trends indicating the percentage to be rising in response to dissatisfaction with managed care restrictions and intrusions.

4. "Please consider that if you have worked hard to become the very best at what you do, and nobody knows, then your capability is irrelevant" (Poynter, 1994, p. 129).

5. "If you are not confident about both your therapeutic and business abilities, you will have a difficult time succeeding in independent practice" (Beigel & Earle, 1990, p. 10).

6. Susan Sturdivant (1990), who wrote some of the early articles on marketing for the American Psychological Association, in noting the lack of consumer knowledge and understanding of what we do, said that if psychotherapy really helps people, then we have a moral and ethical obligation to inform them about our services. She even took it a step further, stating that the most competent therapists (who typically have done the least promoting) must be the

most active marketers or else people will end up choosing the less competent therapists.

3

What Is Marketing?

A DEFINITION OF MARKETING

MARKETING IS AN ATTITUDE
RATHER THAN A "FUNCTION"

In our own terms, it is an effort to "reframe" the practice from the perspective of the provider to that of the consumer. It changes the locus of the practice. It requires that the provider become active in the process of "practice enhancement." It runs counter to what we were taught, which has been referred to as the "Field of Dreams" model; that is, open an office, provide good services, and the patients will come. This, in essence, is a passive model, replete with the anxieties inherent in "waiting for the phone to ring." Marketing provides tools that enable the provider to take active steps to increase the probability that the phone will ring. It also increases the likelihood that the callers are the types of patients you would like to serve. Marketing consists of knowing who you are, where you are going, and how you will get there.

Let me explain what I mean by calling marketing an attitude. It refers to the notion that you are always looking at everything around you in terms of potential to enhance your practice. Things you read, see, or hear can stimulate new ideas. For example, I was reading an article in the town's weekly newspaper about the local real estate association organizing a support program for agents with alcohol problems. I urged our group's substance abuse specialist to contact them, which led to an opportunity to speak and hopefully will produce a new source of referrals. Another article in a Boston paper told me that more police die from suicide than from criminals' bullets. This opened up discussion of a myriad of services that could be offered to local police forces: screening, periodic assessments, marital therapy (due to the unbelievable stress on spouses and children of police officers), and workshops on stress reduction and communication skills.

Whenever there is an announcement of a new physician or attorney opening up in town, we are quick to arrange a meeting and try to establish a relationship. When new guidance counselors or clergy arrive, we do the same. The formation of a new support group is another signal to reach out. All this just comes from reading the local weekly paper and thinking about opportunities to expand your practice. The information is constantly passing in front of you. Articles about trends or needs in the business community (e.g., adults with Attention Deficit Disorder [ADD], diversity training, shyness and its effects on networking, family/work issues, sexual harassment) provide a steady stream of potential ideas that may fit your skills and interests. Please note that many of the latter examples come from one of the best sources of information about what is happening in our field and what opportunities exist for new services: *The Wall Street Journal*. You should read it. The other examples came from local newspapers — both town weeklies and the big city daily. Ideas can come from anywhere; the key is to always be looking.

MARKETING IS EVERYTHING YOU DO
TO PROMOTE YOUR PRACTICE
(Levinson, 1990)

It is not possible to succeed without marketing. You all do it; the questions are whether you are doing it effectively and whether you are achieving the goals you have for your practice.

Word-of-mouth is a marketing strategy — one many of you have lived and died with as your only strategy. The quality of your services, the type of services you offer, and when and where you deliver them are parts of your marketing plan, whether you have actually thought about them or not. Your stationery, clothing, office furnishings, billing system — all are part of the marketing of your practice. How much you read, how often you attend workshops or consult with colleagues, and how you keep your records — all this and more are part of your marketing process. The key question is do you simply do these things haphazardly or are they thought out and put into a format that makes them strategies to achieve the stated goals of your practice? Most of you do the former. After finishing this book, I hope all of you will do the latter.

I have yet to mention advertising. This is the concept most people associate with marketing — and often is the reason mental health professionals avoid learning about marketing. But advertising is simply one item on a list of promotional tactics which, in turn, is but one component of a marketing plan. We will cover advertising and other promotional tactics in later chapters.

Levinson (1990) states that small businesses should "employ with excellence" all the marketing tactics possible — exploit every opportunity. But all the energy, money, and intelligence must have a clear focus, a common purpose, and direction. Note the emphasis on "excellence." The cornerstone of the successful marketing of any independent practice is the quality of your services. If you have no commitment to being the very best clinician you can, then go into another line of work.

One of the advantages of the small businessperson is flexibility. You can shift tactics quickly to take advantage of new ideas or market changes. Thus, despite all the propaganda about the necessity to be part of giant "supergroups," being small (solo or small group) means that you can keep your overhead low, you need only a very small piece of market share, and you can respond to the changing needs of the marketplace much faster than large, bureaucratic systems.

PLANNING

When all is said and done, marketing is really about planning. It not only requires you to think about what you are doing now and about what you hope to do in the future, but it insists that you generate specific, measurable goals and carefully pick strategies that are consistent with those goals. Most importantly, you must write all this down and review it at regular intervals in order to continue to revise your plan until it is working. Two excellent resources to help you understand and carry out the planning aspects of developing and maintaining a practice are *Business Success in Mental Health Practice* (Woody, 1989) and *Managing Your Practice Finances* (American Psychological Association Practice Directorate, 1996).

PROFESSIONAL RESISTANCE TO THE CONCEPT OF OPERATING A BUSINESS

The following discussion is based on Koman (1994).

PSYCHOLOGY IS A HEALING PROFESSION, NOT A BUSINESS: ALTRUISM VERSUS GREED

If you don't make enough money to pay your living expenses, your practice will shut down. Marketing is actually a more socially responsible way to practice because it requires you to think about what the community needs, not just what you feel like doing. It also pushes therapists to be more consumer-friendly (e.g., provide more comfortable seating, be handicapped accessible), to strive to improve the quality of their services, and to seek feedback to find out if their services are effective. So it fits very comfortably with the notion that we are more than just a business and that we have ethical responsibilities as a profession. To take it even further, offering pro bono services or seeing low-fee patients can happen in a planned way and be maintained if you have figured out what net income you need from your practice and how to achieve the latter while offering the former.

WE WEREN'T TRAINED TO DO THIS; WE DIDN'T GO TO BUSINESS SCHOOL

This is one of the more fascinating issues. As a profession, we teach people how to change their behavior. Yet, when we, as a profession, are told we need to change *our* behavior, look at the resistance! Besides, this material is not nearly as complex as most of what we have to learn in order to be competent therapists.

IF IT WEREN'T FOR MANAGED CARE, THIS WOULDN'T BE HAPPENING

Simply not true. In part, this is the natural evolution of a service delivery industry. It is also a response to the concerns about health care costs which are coming from the business world and the federal government. Managed care companies evolved as an opportunistic response to do something about those costs and make a profit from a need. The attitude of blaming managed care for our problems assumes all managed care is bad, which is not true. The emphases on improving quality and demonstrating effectiveness are important positive forces in the current delivery of mental health services. The excesses of managed care are, of course, a serious concern. But as a general concept, accountability should be considered an ethical responsibility.

THE THREE MOST IMPORTANT ELEMENTS OF AN EFFECTIVE MARKETING PROGRAM

The following discussion is based on Levinson (1990).

COMMITMENT

You must take your practice and the concept of marketing seriously. You must have a plan for your practice and keep revising it until it becomes a "powerful plan." You must have patience. Successful marketing is a long-term concept. Once you believe your plan is sound, stick with it, even through hard times. Give it at least 6 months, maybe a year, before changing your strategy. An example is my belief that an ad for a 12-session marital therapy program would be successful in a local monthly newspaper that focuses on parenting. I started running the ad in 1991. During the first year there were only a few calls and the ad lost money. I not only continued to work on improving the design of the ad, but also worked with the paper in terms of placement, encouraging the staff to create a professional directory instead of burying ads like mine among ads for schools and nannies. By the second year the ad began to generate a steady flow of calls, and by 1994, it produced nearly two dozen referrals — a great return on an investment of less than $2,000 per year.

INVESTMENT

Marketing tactics should be considered conservative investments. There is nothing magical or instantaneous here. Effective marketing should result in slow but steady gains over time. The money and time you spend on marketing should be viewed as investing in your practice. Every successful business requires constant reinvestment of some of the revenues in order to continue to improve the business. Therapists traditionally just put the profits in their pockets and then wonder why referrals have dropped off.

CONSISTENCY

You should find an approach that works for *you* and stick with it. Keep yourself and/or your message out there over and over. It is better to run smaller ads more frequently in local papers than periodic big ads in major papers. Similarly, develop a few talks that you can deliver with confidence and ease and seek repeated opportunities to give the talks. Consistency equates with familiarity which leads to referrals. Consistency of marketing reflects confidence in your products and yourself which breeds consumer confidence in you. This means you must choose tactics that you can sustain with the time and/or money that it takes. You need to learn to commit resources for the long term.

THE FIVE BASIC TRUTHS
OF MARKETING

According to Levinson (1993), they are:

1. The market is constantly changing.
2. People forget fast.
3. Your competition isn't quitting.
4. Marketing strengthens your identity.
5. Marketing is essential to survival and growth.

These statements underscore that marketing is not something you do once and it's finished. Marketing is a dynamic process, always being reviewed and refined, requiring a never-ending investment of time and money as long as you desire to maintain a successful practice. For some of us, it also becomes a fun part of the business of private practice. Recently I placed a new ad focusing on services to parents and children. I was not so much motivated by the need for more business as by the fact that I still hadn't found a successful child-oriented ad, and I believe that we should always be looking for ways to strengthen our practice. The paper was offering a special rate, so I wanted to take advantage of the timing, and then there is the challenge of continuously sharpening my marketing skills. I have become as proud of my ability to market my practice as I am of my ability as a therapist. It adds to the joy of my work.

PROFESSIONAL ETHICS

Not very long ago it was unethical to advertise. The Federal Trade Commission (FTC) ordered the American Psychological Association (APA) to change that, but some of our resistance is still embedded in that original but unconstitutional concept. Clearly, if we do advertise, it should not be misleading, false, or deceptive. It is best if it is informative, factual, and educational. Then it serves not only self-promotion but also promotion of the value of mental health services. Other ethical issues that should be addressed as part of developing a business plan include record keeping (including what happens if you die or are incapacitated), informed consent, and risk management. As a good businessperson as well as a good clinician, you need to have studied and developed plans for addressing each of these ethical issues in your practice. Good ethical practices are an essential part of a good business plan. They are not at odds with each other.

4

Service Marketing

In recent years, the field of marketing appears to be evolving from a product marketing orientation to one based on a service marketing approach. The books by Levinson (1990, 1993), for example, are product oriented. They emphasize, as do the later chapters in this book, the four "P"s of marketing: product, price, place, and promotion. A gradual increase in recognition of some unique characeristics in marketing services began about 15 years ago. This shift has expanded into a dramatic turnabout in which newer texts are presenting all businesses as having significant service components that must be reflected in their marketing plan. Service quality and customer satisfaction are seen as the central concepts to be focused on, regardless of the nature of the business. Furthermore, these two factors are intimately linked to all aspects of the business, including operations, financial return, and business vision.

There are four commonly cited characteristics of services that call for different marketing strategies than those for goods (Rust, Zahorik, & Keningham, 1996):

1. **Intangibility:** The most critical difference is that services cannot be seen or touched, only experienced as they

are delivered. Therefore, they are harder to sell because they cannot be examined or tested by the consumer. This means, for our patients, that there is a higher perceived risk in purchasing psychotherapy as compared to an appliance or piece of furniture. The marketing challenge is to provide tangible aids or cues that are reassuring to consumers and increase their confidence in the quality and success of the service. Health care professionals have been notoriously weak in this aspect of servicing consumers. We have paid little attention to educating patients, understanding their perspective of the experience of being a patient, and providing clearer expectations to help them evaluate our services.

2. **Inseparability:** A physical product can stand alone. A "service product" is actually a process that takes place between the provider and the consumer. The interaction between the two parties influences the outcome, which makes it difficult, if not impossible, to standardize the service encounter. This is a direct challenge to attempts to create standard therapy protocols, for no matter how much is scripted, the process from one patient to another will not be the same.

3. **Variability:** An extension of the previous point. Services cannot be consistent and identical, even when delivered by the same provider. It is human nature to be variable: There will be times when you are more alert and focused, and times when you are more tired and less focused. Some patients you will relate to more easily; others will be more discomforting. In theory, efforts to use training to eliminate these variables cannot actually be fully achieved, and even significantly reducing variability may sacrifice the creativity and spontaneity that is essential for the success of the therapy relationship. This once again requires you to recognize that this variability in service performance increases the perceived risk for the patient and requires techniques to reassure patients of the consistency of your commitment to excellence and quality. Many service businesses use guarantees as a very effective means to reassure

their consumers and to insure their own commitment to excellence. In the field of mental health, it may be particularly challenging to offer such guarantees, yet we clearly need to develop ways of reassuring patients and reducing their perception of risk. It may, in fact, be the element of perceived risk, rather than prejudices about receiving mental health services, that prevents so many people from coming to us when they need the services. This may also be why "packaged products," with clearly stated, step-by-step goals and a specific number of sessions, are increasingly popular. It reduces the perception of risk and gives patients the choice of requesting additional services if they have developed confidence in the therapist.

4. **Perishability:** Services are performed in real time; they cannot be inventoried. A service need apears at a given moment and then is gone. Matching capacity to demand is one of the challenges of being an effective provider. Referrals come inconsistently. You can go from being overbooked to having open hours in a short period of time. This causes a lot of stress to therapists. An unused appointment time is revenue lost forever. Even though that time may be used to take care of tasks associated with the delivery of services, if it was meant to be used to see a patient, it cannot be "saved" and "sold" later. However, if you use some of that time for marketing, then the hour's value can be seen as investment in the business, and that does have real dollar value.

Building off these differences between tangible products and intangible services, the four "P"s become seven "P"s by adding people, physical evidence, and process. In this model, "people" refers to the importance of the commitment to excellence by those providing the services. Efforts to generate that commitment are sometimes referred to as "internal marketing." That certainly makes sense, whether it is the solo practitioner pushing himself or herself to take that training program in group therapy or a small group practice committing to weekly peer review sessions. Maintaining a constancy of effort to improve the quality of your services is one of the essentials of building a successful long-term practice. I strongly urge therapists to attend more courses and workshops and to participate in peer consultation. These experiences stimulate professional growth and excitement about your work. They also reduce the potential for burnout.

Physical evidence, referred to as the "serviscape" by Rust et al. (1996, p. 12), pertains to the physical surroundings, the appearance of the provider, and the presence and quality of promotional materials and correspondence. This is often overlooked, but it is very important that the physical evidence support the mission and strategy of the practice. Any such tangible evidence becomes especially significant in helping to assure the patient of the therapist's commitment to quality and, therefore, reducing the patient's sense of risk.

In delivering services, it is not just the final outcome that determines the consumer's subjective evaluation of satisfaction. This is why all aspects of the process — the final "P" — from the initial contact to the final contact and including all aspects of the service operation (billing, waiting time, response to phone calls, etc.) must be dealt with as a series of "moments of truth," each contributing to the patient's experience of your commitment to his or her needs and culminating in a judgment of the degree of satisfaction with your work. It is not necessary that the outcome be successful for the patient to be satisfied. Sometimes an issue does not work out as hoped (a couple who decide to divorce, a child whose school performance doesn't improve, a drug addiction that ends up requiring detox), but the patient is convinced that you did everything expected of you and more even though the situation wasn't salvageable. That patient will walk away telling others how terrific you were and may also return in the future for other services.

The three additional service marketing "P"s are covered in more specific detail in the section of the next chapter that deals with internal assessment and practice operations. It requires an honest evaluation of your strengths and weaknesses as both a therapist and a businessperson and a commitment to excellence in all aspects of your practice. Everything starts with being the most competent therapist possible, but that alone no longer guarantees a successful practice.

Customer satisfaction is the driving force of service marketing. Unlike the patient's perception of the quality of your services, which is a more rational process of evaluating your competence, customer satisfaction is a more subjective, emotional response to how the patient feels about the total service experience. It is greatly influenced by the patient's expectations, which is why sometimes the most difficult patient to satisfy is the one who has heard so many good things about you that he or she starts out with very high expectations. It's comparable to experiences where many friends tell you how great a movie or restaurant is, causing you to expect something phenomenal. Even if the movie or meal is excellent, you often walk away slightly disappointed because you expected even more.

Because customer satisfaction is the primary goal, one of the emerging concepts is called "relationship marketing." It refers to the idea that delivering services or even selling a tangible product should not be viewed as a simple episode where two (or more) people transact some business and it is over. The concept places its emphasis on building a more complex, meaningful, and longer term relationship with the consumer. The original impetus to make this happen comes from the seller (provider) but, gradually, it should be a shared objective with the buyer (patient). It involves looking for ways to be more helpful to the consumer by adding on services or creating an awareness of future ways in which you can be helpful. It means making a greater effort to understand the needs of the patient and how you can help with those needs.

This may be sounding too "businessy," but it is actually very consistent with current concepts of health care and especially mental health services. It means that the provider is trying to establish a long-term relationship that may consist of shorter treatment episodes. It means less emphasis on "terminating" therapy (Have you thought about what a negative-sounding concept that is?) and more emphasis on encouraging patients to return by making that a normal process, not a sign of failure. It recognizes that life is an endless series of chal-

lenges and that it is particularly helpful to have someone to
turn to with a preestablished understanding, connection, and
trust to assist in coping with those challenges. It also recognizes the established business maxim that it costs about five
times more to generate a new customer than it does to keep an
old one.

In many respects, "relationship marketing" is simply establishing yourself as a mental health version of the primary
care physician, an "internist" in a special way of defining "internal"! It fits with Rust et al.'s notion of "reciprocal dependency" (1996, p. 375). Therapists have historically been trained
not to encourage patients to be dependent on them. But, in
typical fashion of being pathologically oriented, the term "dependence" has only a negative, clinical meaning. Instead, consider it similar to the dependence people have on many other
professionals or specialists in their lives: accountants, attorneys, insurance agents, a favorite salesperson in a place you
often shop (partly because of that special relationship), and, of
course, pediatricians and internists. All these service providers remain a constant part of the lives of the consumers, as
long as the providers retain their high rating of customer satisfaction. It is time for mental health professionals to develop a
similar mentality about their relationship to their patients.
Even if you are not always the only therapist providing the
service at different intervals, you can be the person the patient
calls and the one who refers the patient to the specialist that
may be needed at that particular time. This is one reason why
it is important for solo practitioners to have a network of competent colleagues who provide complementary services. This
enables you to remain the central resource as well as being
able to develop a multiple-therapist treatment plan when necessary.

The notion of "retaining patients," one which I have just
begun to focus on, means not only that they return for future
services, but also that they are referring other patients to you
in the future. Developing this concept more fully means considering ways to maintain some form of ongoing contact with
former patients after ending a treatment episode. This can
take the form of an annual mailing to former patients (prob-

ably agreed to by means of a consent form at the end of the first treatment episode) that includes updates on new services you or your associates are offering as well as accomplishments (e.g., papers presented or published, training programs attended). Or it may just be a holiday greeting card wishing that all has continued to go well. The point is to periodically bring you back into the awareness of former patients, which may prompt them to recontact you or to mention you to a friend in need.

As therapists, we may be the ultimate service marketers because our service is a relationship. It is, therefore, of special importance for therapists to understand the unique elements of service marketing and to find ways to incorporate these concepts into their practice.

5

Developing a Business Plan, Part I: Mission Statement, Assessments, and Strategic Vision

A marketing plan is one component of a business plan. The latter typically includes a financial plan, a long-term strategic plan, an operations plan (the logistics of running the business), a human resources plan (staffing), a data management plan, and a statement of goals/tactics for the coming year. It is meant to be a detailed trip map, identifying the business's long-term destination and what is required to get there. Like any trip, there will be unexpected conditions such as bad weather, traffic problems, missed connections, and illness. This means that one must frequently adjust the plan to accommodate these unexpected interferences. A good business plan will also anticipate problems and have contingencies in place (e.g., additional sources of funding if financial projections turn out to be worse than expected). The written plan should be kept as brief as possible, three to five pages. It is a guide, not a detailed text. Woody (1989), Yenney (1994), and "Managing Your Practice Finances" (APA Practice Directorate, 1996) are all excellent resources to help with writing your business plan.

For solo or small group practices, I recommend the following structure for your written business plan:

- **Mission Statement:** The purpose of the practice.
- **Internal Assessment:** Current picture of the practice's strengths and weaknesses (incorporates staffing, operations, and data management).
- **External Assessment:** Current picture of the competition, the business climate, and the needs of the marketplace.
- **Strategic Vision:** 3- to 5-year projection of what the practice should look like, identifying any key changes required to achieve the vision.
- **Specific Goals and Tactics:** Plans for the coming year including measurable goals, dates for achieving the goals, and tactics to be used to achieve the goals.
- **Financials:** Projected income and expenses for the coming year; projected financial needs to achieve strategic vision; methods for financing growth of the business.

This chapter will cover writing a mission statement, completing the internal and external assessments, and creating the strategic vision. Chapter 6 will cover selecting specific goals and tactics and developing a financial plan.

CREATING A MISSION STATEMENT

The mission statement defines the purpose of your practice. Why are you doing this? What do you want to accomplish? What makes your practice unique? What are the primary elements of your practice, and what is the overriding strategy or type of practice? (A list of practice strategies will be presented in Chapter 7.) Where does your practice fit into the rest of your life (family, friends, and other interests, both personal and professional)? Besides therapy services, what other professional activities do you want to do (e.g., teach, write, consult, politics, research, training, public service)?

The length of the mission statement should be kept to a paragraph or two. My current statement reads:

Mission: To maintain a full-time private practice of the highest quality, enhancing my image as an expert in the fields of child development, marriage, and family; to increase alternative income sources (nonpatient); to increase my professional writing; to continue to contribute to the development of Needham Psychotherapy Associates as a successful group practice; and to continue to maintain a healthy balance of family life, travel, and outside interests (stocks, sports, and community service).

This mission statement provides me with a constant guiding light to help make sure I am using my time properly and creates the context for developing more specific marketing goals.

Take a break from reading and write a rough draft of your practice mission. Share it with a colleague for some feedback and return to it when you have finished the book for a final version which will be the opening section of your first marketing plan. Appendix A (pp. 129-132) contains several sample mission statements tied to specific goals and strategies.

INTERNAL ASSESSMENT

This part of your business plan requires that you thoroughly analze your practice, including your office, record keeping, equipment, interactions with patients, interactions with referral sources and the community, professional development, money management, and emotional management (psychotherapy is an intense interpersonal process). You will probably want to seek feedback from colleagues, family, and friends in order to get an accurate picture of all the elements. This is the part that I referred to in the previous chapter as incorporating the three special components of service marketing: people, physical evidence, and process.

Many details contribute to a successful practice. You need to look at emergency coverage, coverage when you are away, use of clerical support, your location, accessibility of your office, sense of confidentiality (sound management), furnishings (Is there comfortable seating; is it a warm, soothing setting?), your waiting room (check comfort, reading materials, privacy), your cards and stationery, and use of books and tapes to supple-

ment your work. A broader question: Do you present yourself
as a professional in your dress, manner, setting, and style? Your
financial management has to do with paying your business bills,
keeping good records for tax purposes, having a good accountant, and maintaining adequate insurance coverage. As a self-
employed person, you need to develop your own benefits package: health insurance, life insurance, disability insurance, of-
fice/injury insurance, office overhead (a must — it's a great
bargain and great protection), and, of course, malpractice insurance. Equally important is retirement planning. Do you
know about the different formats for tax-protected retirement
plans, and have you spent some time understanding how your
money should be invested? If you are deficient in any of these
areas, seek colleagues or consultants who can help you. Lenson
(1994) and Yenney (1994) are especially helpful in covering all
the details of operating a practice.

More questions to ask yourself: What type of patients do
you like to work with? What types of problems are you best at
solving? Have you developed a strong presence in your community? Do you maintain frequent face-to-face contact with
your primary referral sources? It's amazing that for people
who are in the relationship business, we often do a lousy job of
cultivating the important relationships we need to be successful!

How do you promote yourself? Do you distribute copies of
articles you've published? Do you keep information about your
practice in the waiting room? Some people ask, "Why bother?
These are already my patients." Keeping brochures, copies of
articles, and press releases in your waiting room helps to confirm the decisions of new patients and reaffirms the confidence
of continuing patients (an important aspect of reducing the
sense of perceived risk in their purchase of your services). It
tells your patients and your colleagues' patients (if you share a
waiting room) about specialty services you offer and may lead
them to make referrals. I have often found that my own patients don't know about certain services I offer. That's why
keeping your own brochure in your waiting room is good marketing and contributes to effective treatment. Psychotherapy
research increasingly points to the significance of the patient's

belief in your framework for explaining their problems as a critical factor in successful outcomes (part of the reason why many different approaches are successful). Therefore, whatever you do that contributes to a patient having more confidence in you as a competent professional will contribute to positive outcomes.

You also need handouts that clarify how you run your practice, payment procedures, and informed-consent and release-of-information forms. All this needs to be covered in your initial session, which may mean you need to allow extra time for the business aspects of creating a therapeutic alliance.

All this leads to a discussion of what I consider to be the four critical operational elements of a successful practice: initial response to a referral, money, quality of services, and records.

INITIAL RESPONSE TO A REFERRAL

How quickly do you respond? Do you allow time to make a real connection with the patient on the phone, and is the first appointment scheduled within their "time need"? Remember, you are selling yourself. Even if prospective patients cannot see me (due to insurance, time, or specialty treatment needs), I make a point of assisting them in finding a competent therapist who can serve them. I try to never require a patient to have to make a second phone call. Making that first one is hard enough. So I will call the prospective therapist and have that person call the patient. The reason I invest the time in doing this is that patients, even if they can't get to see me, will be a potential source of referrals in the future, and it is consistent with my commitment to helping to insure that people who call me end up with the best possible services.

I use an intake card that insures that I collect all necessary information in one place. The card is thick and specially colored for easy access. Consistent with the notion that I am in part selling a service in that phone call, I believe it is very important to "close" the referral by getting the patient to commit to an appointment time. Patients who need to think it over or talk to a spouse frequently do not call back. When I follow up with a return call, often the person has decided to put off getting help. When patients make that first call, they are at their maximum level of motivation to initiate help. If I can get them to schedule an appointment, with the option of canceling if they change their mind, they are more likely to come in. The time I invest in patients in that initial phone call pays off. I have very few no-shows and very few patients who show once and never return.

I recommend using answering machines or voice mail because these allow for more detailed, confidential information to be left and reduce errors. Pagers can be used for emergencies. Be sure to call or write referral sources to say thanks, to clarify what their concerns are, and to agree on what feedback they want.

MONEY

This is one of our most serious weaknesses as business-people. We tend to avoid the issue. You need to be very clear up front about how much you charge and what you charge for (telephone time; travel time for school, home, or other consultations; report writing; computerized testing; reviewing of written records or reports from other professionals). We tend to give away too much of our time. As I mentioned earlier, we need to consider ourselves professionals and value our services and time. If we don't, why should the patient?

Do you explain your billing procedures? A handout describing fees, billing procedures, insurance procedures, and practice policies is an essential part of your initial session. (Zuckerman [1997] is an excellent resource for all the forms you might use in your practice.) You need to have an effective system for billing and bring up failure to pay when any month passes without a payment. Try, whenever possible, to collect fees at each session. The use of credit cards is slowly increasing. If patients end treatment with an outstanding balance, it may become difficult to collect. Using collection agencies or attorneys is not very desirable, and small-claims court takes up your valuable time. The cheapest way is *to keep your collections up to date.*

In today's managed care environment, it is especially important to review insurance coverage in detail. Strongly encourage patients to familiarize themselves with their plan's requirements, payments, and limits. Patients must realize their responsibility to pay for services in case certification/payment is denied. It is also essential to discuss confidentiality issues related to third-party payments, because we are often required to share extensive information with managed care companies (MCCs) in order to get approval for coverage. Patients need to understand this and make a knowledgeable decision about using their insurance as opposed to paying out of pocket.

QUALITY OF SERVICES

Quality is always the cornerstone of a successful practice/ business. But you must understand that it is the "perceived quality" that counts — that is, what your patient's experience or perception is of the services being received. This is one of the most frequently overlooked and misunderstood issues. It requires knowing what patients want from you, integrating their expectations with your own assessment of what the problem is, and arriving at a set of common goals. A realistic and shared vision of what to expect from therapy is essential to successful outcomes.

Quality service also means allowing adequate time for appointments and returning phone calls. Don't make patients feel as if they are being rushed through a treatment assembly line. A sense of caring must be cultivated. Never, never answer your phone during sessions! Don't schedule patients back-to-back with no time between appointments. That's not only greedy, it shows that quality is not your priority. You can't complete your notes, return important calls, or allow your own emotional recovery or reflection to take place.

A commitment to quality services also means a strong investment in continuing education. Do you make time to read journals and books? Do you attend effective workshops? (The operative word is "effective"; select programs that are intensive enough to actually result in improving your old skills or in learning new ones; the latter means committing significant resources, time, and money — nobody learns a new treatment technique from a few hours of lectures.) This becomes especially critical if you have decided that one of your business goals is to develop a new service, for example, neuropsychological testing, custody evaluations, or biofeedback.

RECORDS

Keeping good notes is not only an ethical and, in many states, a legal requirement, but essential to careful thought and ongoing assessment of what you are doing. It is also a must for risk management (malpractice outcomes are often determined by adequacy of records). Good record keeping also means having in place a plan for what happens to your records (and your patients) if you die or become incapacitated. Be aware that patients can sue your estate if this is not properly handled and confidentiality is broken or patients' needs are not provided for according to current standards of practice.

Record keeping includes collecting patient feedback and outcome data. Keep it very simple — global assessment of functioning (GAF) scores or a symptom checklist are sufficient for evaluating clinical outcomes. A short list of questions — no more than a page or two, designed so the answers can be quantified — should be administered at the end of therapy and in at least one follow-up, for example, at 6 months, which can be done randomly or routinely. It is probably best if the patient satisfaction survey is done on the telephone and not by the therapist (because of the many complex relationship issues that can affect what the patient would say). Typically, for a small practice, your secretary would conduct the survey in order to allay concerns about confidentiality.

Records should also show summaries of information about your patients (towns, ages, diagnoses, length of treatment) and your referral sources. This allows analysis of your practice (business) in order to figure out what changes may be needed to improve business or simply enjoy it more (e.g., balance of different diagnoses).

In addition to these four cornerstones of an effective practice, internal assessment requires that you examine the technology of your practice: owning a computer, fax machine, and copier. Do you use a computerized billing program? An office management system that keeps track of referrals, notes, and expenses? Computerized testing? Desktop publishing? Are you ready for online billing? Do you have an E-mail address? A Web site? Do you use the Internet? Technology, especially owning a computer, is becoming so essential to good practice that I may soon call it the fifth cornerstone of an effective practice.

An important component in managing a successful practice is a good secretary. Yes, even a solo practitioner operating out of a home office should invest in a good part-time secretary. Your time is too valuable to be spent doing secretarial tasks (this is not to demean the secretary's value, which is enormous); in addition, the secretary will develop specialty knowledge about dealing with insurance companies or managing press releases or running a billing program or word processing program that you just don't have the time (or inclination) to do. The secretary may also be a good source of community information, can do research for you, and, if you have the equipment, can do desktop publishing, which can be a real money saver when it comes to promotional activities. One of the most important issues in hiring a good secretary is to insure an understanding of the special nature of the confidentiality of your work. This is especially critical if the secretary is doing the work at home. You must see for yourself how materials are protected from the eyes of anyone else.

In the final analysis, internal assessment means identifying where your practice is strong and weak and integrating that information into your business plan. This means planning how to get the maximum utilization out of your strengths in order to achieve the goals you have set. In fact, the goals should reflect your strengths. In addition, you must also identify the ways in which your weaknesses may be impeding the success of your practice and plan ways to reduce those negative effects.

EXTERNAL ASSESSMENT

Of all the components of a business plan for a private practice, this is probably the one that has changed the most, is still changing the most, and the one you have the least control over, the least understanding of, and the least likelihood of being able to predict. The soothsayers claim it is the external factors — in particular, managed care in its various forms — that will determine who will provide what kinds of services in what kinds of settings. In other words, "they" are saying you will have a very limited role in determining your future as a health care provider, and your primary option is to become part of some larger system and follow their rules. The problem is that no one has ever been very successful at predicting behavior or business trends. Everyone relies on linear models and just draws straight lines out to some apparently logical conclusion. But life does not operate in a linear fashion. Typically, as forces move in a certain direction, new forces develop that did not even exist before and the whole process moves toward a different "trend," then another trend, and so on. Also, the entire country, even single states, appears to be experiencing very different patterns of practice in different areas. The concepts of group contracts, supergroups, outcomes research, vertically integrated systems, and capitation are all developing in much more uneven and uncertain fashion than the industry leaders keep predicting. This doesn't mean that managed care is not going to change the face of health care, especially mental health care. But the way it will do this, the timetable for it, and what choices you have to make are much less predictable than the headlines would suggest.

Following are a few examples of what I mean. Recently I read that only about 20% of managed care companies are actually collecting outcomes data, and they are discovering it is a very expensive process. This will alter what gets done — and when. Also, referrals to supergroups are not developing as quickly as expected in some of the geographic areas where they have been strongly promoted (e.g., California and Minnesota). In the Greater Boston area, contracts with groups are moving very slowly. Plus, the concept of pushing everything toward provider-based capitation is being rethought by MCCs, because that might eliminate the need for MCCs if they are not assuming any risk! Furthermore, there is always the possibility that state or federal legislation could alter what MCCs can or must do. In addition, if the point-of-service option (being able to choose providers not on the panel for a higher deductible and a higher copayment) continues to increase significantly, the impact of managed care will be reduced for those currently shut out of panels. Likewise, "any willing provider" legislation has been passed in several states, which also reduces the restrictions on which patients you can serve, though it still results in reduced fees and added paperwork.

All this means that you must stay informed of national and local changes and decide whom you are going to believe about fuure trends. Then you must decide how much your practice will be shaped according to both external and internal factors (see Chapter 7 about choosing a practice strategy).

In addition to the impact of managed care, there are other external factors that should be considered, such as population trends, locally and nationally. For example, despite the alleged prominence of nontraditional families, there are communities in the Greater Boston area in which tradition reigns supreme. Promoting services to single-parent families in towns where over 90% of the families have intact marriages is probably not a successful strategy! There is also a "bump" in the population of children which has been packing overcrowded elementary schools for the past few years and will soon lead to a surge in adolescents. This should generate potential services related to those age groups. Of course, we are all familiar with the "graying of America" as people live longer and are more active and productive into their senior years; this population will gradually be bolstered by the arrival of the aging "baby boomers," a highly educated and relatively affluent group who have a positive investment in the value of psychotherapy.

The key with demographics is understanding your target community. How culturally diverse is it? What do you need to learn to serve your community? Are different types of services required in urban centers or rural communities?

Beyond demographics, one always needs to analyze the competition. Who is your competition? These days you are facing an increasing range of options as both general and psychiatric hospitals develop outpatient services — this in addition to the usual solo and group practices and, to a lessening degree, publicly funded programs. You not only need to understand the "who" but also the "what"; that is, what types of services are being offered in what formats and for what fees. There appears to be a major emphasis on the concept of vertically integrated services. This refers to offering a full range of outpatient, partial care, and inpatient services all within a single organization in order to provide "seamless" (one of the new hot words) services. But we don't know if the typical outpatient consumer cares about or needs this type of organization, which is much more expensive to operate than a private practice and, inevitably, more impersonal and bureaucratic. However, some MCCs are developing contracts with these hospital-based organizations, which would reduce their need for provider panels.

You must be knowledgeable about the managed care companies that are major forces in your community, whether you seek to be on their panels or not. This will help you develop your skills at dealing with insurance companies, HMOs, and preferred provider organizations (PPOs). Much of that information can be found in your local newspapers. In addition, there are several newsletters that try to keep you up to date on who's buying out whom, what the very latest trends are, and the most recent news from state and federal governments. A list of these resources will be found in Appendix B (pp. 133-134). Poynter (1994) is probably the best single resource for advice on how to try to get on panels and how to develop effective working relationships with MCCs. C. Browning and B. Browning's (1994) *How to Partner with Managed Care* is also excellent.

Just another comment about trends. In nearly every industry, especially those that require more modest capital investment, the business goes through a period in which "bigger is better," the so-called industry shake-out, when, allegedly, only the strong survive. The inefficiencies of bureaucracy then allow many small businesses to emerge successfully, either because they can better serve certain niche markets or because they just better serve their customers. So listen with some skepticism to the idea that small mental health businesses are doomed. Keep in mind that the majority of Americans work for small businesses, not large corporations. That number actually seems to be increasing: The younger generation has a strong entrepreneurial attitude, partly because big companies have lost their loyalty to their employees and no longer offer the advantage of job security.

Nevertheless, five or six large companies will soon own 90% of the health care marketplace and will have the major say in shaping the rules of the game. During this process, I expect most of the current HMOs and PPOs to go out of business by purchase, merger, or failure. Ultimately, the insurance companies will see that it is much more profitable to eliminate the extra layer of cost, namely MCCs. But managed care will probably be the way they require business to be done because their clients, the corporations who purchase health care policies, want cost containment.

It's not very clear what the corporations will continue to insist upon in terms of costs and services. As more data get published showing the devastating cost of mental health disorders in the workplace through absenteeism and diminished performance, corporations could become our strongest allies in pushing for the equality of mental and medical health care. But we don't know if mental health care will continue to be included in future legislative changes, much less whether it will achieve parity of coverage. What we must do is continue to fund our professional organizations' efforts to represent us and to insist they do so wisely by our staying informed and becoming more politically active. We also need to seek ways of being less divided by discipline, because our intra-turf warfare makes us much less able to fight for mental health care in the marketplace and political arenas.

It is important to be knowledgeable about what is going on around us. Through the combination of understanding our own strengths and weaknesses and being informed about our competition and the external forces that impact on us, we can develop a strategy for our practice that will have a maximum probability of being successful.

STRATEGIC VISION

This section focuses on intermediate goals. In certain respects, this is the real driving force behind your efforts to change the way you practice. Your vision of what you hope to be doing in a few years will determine much of your specific goal-oriented activities during the next 12 months. For example, if your vision is that in 5 years you would like to derive one-third of your income from divorce mediation as a natural extension of your large marital therapy practice, you might plan the following sequence:

- **First Year:** Talk to therapists in the area already doing mediation; find out the pros and cons of going into that work, what kind of training is required to be considered well-prepared, and what costs are associated with the training and the start-up of a new part of your practice.
- **Second Year:** Assuming the information gathered is positive, this would be the training year (or maybe it would take 2 years of training). How would you deal with the time and expense demands of this training?
- **Third Year:** What promotional tactics would be used to make people aware of your new skills and how could you generate referrals? How would you obtain continued supervision until you had enough experience to feel comfortable doing it on your own?

This model can be duplicated for any number of professional goals, ranging from new clinical skills to adding new dimensions to your professional life such as teaching, research, political activism, or writing a book. The important concept is that you must always be taking a longer view of your career, because if you don't plan for these changes, they won't happen. Equally important is the self-questioning — the internal analysis — that should be an ongoing part of your career: Do you really love what you are doing? Are there other professional (or nonprofessional) activities that you want to be doing in the future? What are the marketplace trends, and how can you best take advantage of them? Always check your strategic vision against your mission to make sure you aren't going off in directions inconsistent with your reasons for being in practice. Opportunities often present themselves that are tempting but may detract from your primary career goals. Similarly, you must also test your strategic vision against the information found in the internal and external assessments. Does this really fit with your skills? Does it mesh with the existing structure of the practice? By the time you are ready to do this, will the marketplace need you? This is why strategic planning comes as the fourth step in the process.

An example from my group practice ties together the previous sections and segues into the remainder of the book. Our group determined that part of its mission was to try to become the dominant mental health provider in the local community. We tried to create an objective definition to this vision which included a significant increase in the number of patients who lived in the community. The timeline to achieve this was 5 years. We recognized that among many strategies involved in trying to accomplish this vision was to create closer working relationships with the medical community and the school system. We began a process that has included increased involvement with the community hospital, regular mailings to and meetings with local physicians, offering in-service workshops to the school staff, becoming involved with special projects in the school system, and regular meetings with various school personnel.

Over the past 2 years, we can see a steady increase in the number of physicians referring to us, the number of referrals from the school system, and the number of local patients. As we track the progress, we annually review what seems to work and what doesn't. Also, unexpected opportunities always pop up. Remember, marketing is an attitude, and you must always be looking for new possibilities. We can see that we are moving in the right direction and that the process is gaining momentum. But there is still much to be done; success is by no means guaranteed. The key is that we had a clear vision and we have constantly used that vision to determine where to place our resources.

6

Developing a Business Plan, Part II: Marketing Plan And Financials

THE MARKETING PLAN

The marketing plan is a statement of specific objectives for your practice in the coming year and what tactics will be used to achieve those goals. Tactics and promotional options will be covered in Chapters 8 to 10. For now, we will focus on setting goals and planning funding.

The objectives evolve from your mission statement and the strategic vision of your practice. They should have some measurable component that makes evaluation easier, for example, to increase general referrals by a certain number, to develop a certain amount of revenue from a new activity, or to increase net after-tax profits by a certain amount. Net after-tax profit simply refers to what is left when you subtract the cost of running your practice from your gross income, including income taxes paid on the pre-tax, adjusted gross income. Adjusted gross income refers to your gross income minus your business expenses.

Goals may reflect the number of patients you want to see in an average week, the types of patients, the hours of your practice, the time and money you are devoting to marketing, and specific nonpatient, professional activities that you would like to develop as sources of income. For example, 4 years ago I decided that my strategy in a market heavily penetrated by HMOs would be to focus on promoting directly to the public (as opposed to referral sources or managed care companies). Given that approximately one-third of all callers might be ineligible to be reimbursed for my services, I set a goal of raising my rate of referrals from four to six per month and then increased that goal to seven because of the increased emphasis on short-term clinical work that even the public is very conscious of these days. My tactics included more advertising, developing a couple of specialty products, creating a new brochure, significantly increasing the number of lectures, expanding the publication of my newspaper column on parenting, and trying to get some articles published in other local newspapers and magazines. I considered a program for my local cablevision but decided I didn't have the time. However, I drafted a few ideas for possible future use.

Most of the tactics were utilized as planned, some I still haven't gotten to (e.g., magazine publication), and some of the advertising dollars were not effectively spent. It took 2 years to achieve the rate-of-referral goal. Now I have exceeded it in the past 2 years. That's one of the great benefits of a successful marketing program: Once rolling, its momentum increases, partly because satisfied patients are still the best referral base, and that base just keeps growing.

Marketing goals typically include:

1. **Profitability:** This requires us to look at what percentage of our gross is needed to cover expenses; is it too high (or not high enough)? According to a recent *Psychotherapy Finances* survey ("Fee, Practice," 1995),*

---

*By the way, the annual survey by *Psychotherapy Finances* ("Fee, Practice," 1995) is a wonderful source of information about the trends in our field. This issue showed that direct pay and traditional insurance still accounted for two-thirds of private practice income, that there has been an increase in therapists offering evening and weekend hours, and that three-fourths of the 1,700 therapists surveyed are still solo practitioners. But group practices are growing in number and show a definite trend toward shorter therapy (a mean of 15.6 sessions vs. 21.3 for solo practitioners). This helps you to understand the competition and where you fit into the professional trends.

the median overhead is 32%, regardless of type of practice. My own was approximately 29% in 1996, so I am managing my costs fairly well despite significant spending on ads and brochures. Check your figures. You should also know your average revenue per patient hour — a key statistic. Mine is $92, against a current top fee of $120. When you multiply this average by your actual net profit percentage (100 - .29 = .71), the result is your actual pre-tax profit per patient hour ($92 x .71 = $65.32 per session). This formula helps you determine how many patients you need to see in order to achieve annual revenue goals. If it doesn't work, then you need to look at ways to reduce costs, increase fees, or develop other sources of revenue. By setting goals, instead of operating on some vague notion of making a living, this process requires you to know what you are actually making. If your business isn't successful, it will lead you to change goals or strategies in order to be sufficiently profitable.

An analysis of profitability provides the base for making many decisions about your practice. Do you need to reduce overhead, raise fees, or generate other sources of income? Can you afford new equipment or to increase the hours of your secretary? Too many therapists make these decisions without the necessary information.

2. **Sales (Revenue) Growth:** This is a tough one for therapists. The primary ways to increase revenues are to see more patients or raise fees. If you are generally booked and don't want to increase your hours, and if the local economy inhibits raising your fees, your income stagnates. Even worse, the more managed care infiltrates your practice, your average fee per session may drop and your income may actually decrease — even, in some cases, where the number of patients has increased.

Thus you may need alternative strategies to increase your revenues. These would primarily include increasing the percentage of full-fee patients (Do you know what that percentage is now?), conducting psycho-ed groups, offering services to corporations (e.g., wellness seminars, executive coaching), doing forensic work or custody evaluations, or offering workshops for a fee (e.g., parenting, stress management, marital). Again, the issue in developing a marketing plan is to generate a clear picture of your practice and to evolve strategies to fix the problem areas.

3. **Market Share Improvement:** If your available patient hours are not full, then you need more referrals in order to have more patients. In business terms, this is called increasing market share, which simply means you want to increase your percentage of the mental health business coming from your target communities (geographic, diagnostic, and age groups).

First, you need to determine who are the target populations for your practice. Start by using the data from your internal assessment about where your current and past patients have come from — by location, by referral source, and by diagnosis. Decide if the result matches the desired profile of your practice. In reviewing this, you must also consider if the populations you are seeking to treat and the services you wish to offer are really in demand in your area. Then think about which of these you would like to set goals to increase. For this discussion, let's say that, based on demographic data (most states can provide profiles on towns) and research on rates of different diagnostic categories, your community probably has a potential of 2,000 mental health referrals annually and you are getting only 20. You have only 1% of that market share. If you double your market share to 2%, or 40 referrals, that may be sufficient to fill your open slots. That leads to a set of strategies on how to become better known in your immediate geographic area and an ability to measure whether you are being successful in your efforts. This goal doesn't sound so overwhelming when you realize how small a piece of the marketplace you need to be successful. (The tactics to achieve these goals will be presented in Chapters 8, 9, and 10.)

Please understand that estimating the number of potential annual referrals in your target community is highly speculative and that small practices don't usually think in terms of market share. I use this example just to stress the potential business that exists right in your backyard. In all likelihood, you will use other indices to measure your practice's growth, such as revenue and number of referrals.

Of course, you may also target market "segments" or marketing niches, which refers to more narrow target groups. This can be a diagnostic category (ADHD, bi-polar disorders, phobias), particular life problems (cardiac recovery patients, divorce support, job loss), special age groups (infants and toddlers, geriatrics, teens), or more focused geographic targets (high-income neighborhoods with the goal of getting more cash patients). One idea for targeting specific neighborhoods is a small newsletter, with some brief articles about mental health issues and treatments, mailed two to four times per year, only to the more affluent sections of your town.

4. **Budget (Money and Time):** Marketing requires a real commitment. It must be a regular part of your work week and must be part of your business expenses. Thus, in developing your marketing plan you must figure out how much time and money you are designating for your marketing efforts and try to determine if it is sufficient to achieve the goals that you have set and the tactics that you have chosen. It is generally recommended that 10% to 15% of your income (figuring the value of your time as well as direct expenditures) be committed to your marketing efforts. More appropriate than a rule of thumb, however, is setting marketing priorities, figuring out what it may cost to achieve those goals, and then figuring out if you can afford the cost. Then you manipulate costs by selecting less expensive tactics or by eliminating other expenses from your budget if you decide this must be done in a particular way or not at all. As you read over and over, marketing is about planning.

As an example of what a statement of goals may look like, here is the list from my current marketing plan:

> To expand my marketing workshop product; to develop marketing consultation services; to find a second ad that generates referrals; to expand my exposure through writing (column published in more towns or other publications, articles published in professional or lay publications); to give more lectures; to maintain current level of referrals (7-8/mo.); to explore Alternative Dispute Resolution as a possible new income source; to increase frequency of corporate workshops to 2-3/mo.; switch to a new version of my billing program; develop a personal, generic brochure; begin to collect better patient data (# of sessions, outcome); and continue to assist Needham Psychotherapy Associates in increasing referrals to the group and developing a relationship to a vertically integrated, hospital based system.

Take another reading break and develop a list of goals for your practice. As always, it helps to review them with a colleague and to make revisions after completing the book.

FINANCIAL PLANNING

Although a mental health practice requires much less capitalization than most other small businesses, do not underestimate the need for adequate capital. You must purchase necessary equipment, select quality furnishings, and have an office that is properly located and attractive, not only for your patients but also as a place to work. You need money for promotional materials, proper insurance coverage, and competent legal, accounting, and financial advice. In addition, you must have continued access to capital as needed for refurbishing, purchasing new equipment, attending out-of-town conferences, or taking expensive training programs to develop new skills for a private practice. This means you must sit down and figure out how much you need to get started or how much you need to maintain a quality practice. It means knowing your costs and your after-tax profits.

It also means integrating your practice income into your family financial planning. For some, private practice income is a small piece of the family income. In these situations, sometimes there's less willingness (or support) to invest more in the practice. For others in an identical situation, there is support to invest more and take greater risks toward hoped-for, longer-term rewards. This is particularly true for therapists who plan to expand their practices as their children get older. I cannot stress often enough the value of planning. One of the frequent mistakes I see is part-time therapists not taking their practice seriously and forever complaining about how unsuccessful it is. You must be committed to doing everything with competence — the maximum competence that you can bring to the situation. Anything less, particularly in the current tumultuous and competitive marketplace, is likely to keep you in a rut of mediocrity. Which brings us back to the importance of financial planning. Most businesses die for lack of funds. Don't make this mistake. Make sure you are setting aside part of your profits to reinvest in the business, and make sure you have access to emergency sources of capital if needed.

7

Selecting a
Practice Strategy

The concept of practice strategies was first described to me in a workshop led by Monica Oss in 1990. Though some of the details and choices have changed over time, the basic concept remains valid. Every practice, be it solo or group, needs to define its primary way of achieving its mission. Just as every successful company can be described in terms of its "culture," so must your practice be defined by its primary strategy. Of course, some of these strategies may be combined, but you still must have a clear vision or else the decisions you make about allocating resources will lack a focus, resulting in considerable inefficiency and less likelihood of success.

EIGHT STRATEGIES
FOR SUCCESS

SPECIALIZATION

Specialization means pursuing a specific market niche, developing services that are sensitive to the needs of a well-defined target group (a segment of a community, a specific disorder, a group sharing a common life situation), and providing services that are *perceived* as better and more desirable than those of your competitors. Occasionally you may even be able to develop a niche that lacks competition, though that won't last long once the word gets around. Selection of the target is critical. It must have potential for revenue, profit, and growth. That means there must be a need for the services, a receptivity for the services, and a lack of significant competition — unless you have a unique concept that would give you a competitive advantage. This is a good strategy for a solo or small group practice. In fact, it is the essential strategy for the solo practitioner unless you are famous or so well-established that you don't even need to be reading this! The rule of thumb is that the smaller you are, the more you need to specialize. In a small business you don't need so many referrals, promotion is more efficient (your resources are limited), and, once established, you can often charge premium prices because you have established yourself as an expert. Don't be afraid of getting only one type of patient. As people get to know you through this model, they will send you other referrals (if you are competent). Risks: Misreading the need, not promoting effectively, or failing to keep up with evolving knowledge in the specialty.

Again, specialization is one of the best concepts for solo and small group practitioners. You don't have to change your basic practice; the niche may even be something you already do but have never refined into a clinical "product." My personal example of this is "Marital Enhancement Therapy," a 12-session marital therapy program. I simply formalized what I had been doing for many years (marital therapy rooted in Virginia Satir's seminal work with a strong developmental component and a dash of contemporary gender role and communication analysis), developed a brochure and an ad, and my marital therapy business has tripled. Meanwhile, the ad has prompted calls for services not even listed — including a call from a work/family consulting company. I now lead several corporate workshops annually because of that phone call. It's part of the basic concept of marketing that, if you get your name out there on a regular basis, good things will begin to happen, some of them unpredictable.

Psychotherapy Finances has recognized the high value of specialization; they call it "niche marketing." In addition to providing their original list of the top 40 practice niches ("Forty Practice Niches," 1995) — the top five being medical rehabilitation, disease management, pain control/stress management, disabled population, and gero-psychiatric — they publish niche-marketing articles in virtually every issue. Two of those articles provide excellent examples ("Niche Marketing," 1995). The first described a therapist who developed a specialty in services for women in their late 30s who had put off having children and then experienced fertility problems. She started by researching the topic (so important — the cornerstone is always competence) and then developed a marketing plan. Her efforts resulted in achieving her goal of seeing 14 infertility patients per week within 10 months. A side benefit is that two-thirds are paying out of pocket (not unusual if there is no competition and you are very good at what you do). She even got onto "closed" panels because nobody else was providing this service.

The second niche was working with hearing-impaired clients (note: both these therapists chose their niches based on personal experiences with the problem). This is an area of substantial need in our communities and would be especially helped by any therapist willing to invest in learning sign language. This therapist ended up with a group practice and hospitals clamoring for his services.

As reflected in these examples, the specialty strategy will usually draw a higher percentage of out-of-pocket payers and increase your income while reducing your reliance on third-party payers. In addition, if the specialty is attractive to MCCs, they may place you on their otherwise-closed panel just for that particular service. There will be more discussion about developing specialties in Chapter 8 when I discuss mental health "products."

QUALITY LEADER; THE "EXPERT"

It is not just the actual clinical quality of your services but the perceived quality that counts in this model. You can charge premium prices because you are known as "the" person to go to for this problem. It's an easy marketing message to communicate, but you must have the special credentials that your target groups will easily relate to (e.g., top university or hospital affiliation, publications, and special awards that clearly establish you as one of the top people in this segment of the market). Second only to writing a best-seller in effectiveness, this strategy usually takes time to develop and tends to fit experienced practitioners who have developed their reputation over the years. This strategy is similar to specialization, because if you successfully develop a specialty you are likely to be perceived as an expert in that service.

Public relations is an important part of this strategy. Experts are usually the people who appear on the local talk shows, are interviewed for important newspaper articles, and headline large workshops. There are few risks other than becoming dated and getting pushed aside by rising, new experts. The difficulty is achieving the status to begin with. Quality leaders usually have a higher percentage of cash payers and are often able to choose to minimize involvement with panels.

LOW PRICE LEADER

This refers to "acceptable" quality services at a low market price. The focus is on a high-volume, low-cost approach, which typically makes use of lower fee staff. Obtain contracts to ensure volume. Develop innovative models. Because this is more of a "business" model, it may be less attractive to small practices. Advantages include potential to dominate a market, larger profit potential, and entrepreneurial satisfaction. Risks are higher because of staffing and contract commitments, the capital investment required, and narrow profit margin. You can hit it big — or take a bath! This model fits the current strategies of the managed care companies, so it is opportunistic.

ECLECTIC STRATEGY

Closer to what most of us have been doing, this is a middle-ground position, trying to provide a variety of good quality services at reasonable costs and to create a perception of "good value." Try to control costs. Try to stay current in techniques. Offer a range of services in order to try to fit the needs of a wide range of patients. In today's marketplace, this is a very risky strategy, because you may not be able to differentiate yourself from the competition, and your practice could die a slow death. If you are well-established, you may have enough momentum to last through the shake-out and see what the playing field looks like. But I would recommend some accommodations to the current market by combining this with one of the other strategies or making a much greater commitment to promotion. Also make sure you are operating a financially efficient practice.

TECHNOLOGY LEADER

This growing aspect of our business includes using computers for intake, testing, records, case monitoring, outcomes data, and electronic billing. Telephone therapy! Limo Therapy! Using the Internet. Being on the Internet. Biofeedback. EEG (for ADHD). Light therapy for treating seasonal affective disorder (SAD). In other words, use any form of equipment-based technology to create specialized treatments or to just operate a more high-tech practice. This strategy calls to mind the early years of family therapy when video was integrated into treatment — only now it is the computer and not the video camera that must be mastered.

The newest phase of technological development is the Internet. This electronic highway connects you to an incredible array of people and services. It offers many current and future possibilities that may ultimately have a significant impact on the way we practice. A recent survey (Kalfel, 1996) points out some of these trends. In 1995, personal computers outsold TVs for the first time. The majority of people in the survey who had decided to seek mental health services conducted some research about their problem before making a call. The average "surfer" comes from a well-educated family with an average income of $70,000. Add to this the explosion in subscriptions to online services and the impending integration of TV, cable, and the Internet. It doesn't take much of a fantasy to imagine incredible new ways to interact with a public which has always struggled to comprehend mental health problems and services.

Creating a Web site for your practice beats the Yellow Pages in every way imaginable — and it's cheaper, after the initial set-up costs. A Web site offers far more information, such as pictures and bios of all therapists, copies of published articles, chat rooms where questions can be answered before meeting, and referral services to other helpful Web sites or to other practitioners. You can provide regular updates on new services and on workshops. All this and *it is interactive!* Certainly there is tremendous potential for the Internet and the World Wide Web to be an incredible marketing opportunity for practitioners and the mental health field. You can create your own Web site with software or hire a consultant to set up your page as well as teach you how to get the most out of it.

But the Internet is not just for patients. Therapists can access articles of interest as well as chat with professionals around the world about challenging clinical questions. It is possible that the long delays between generating helpful research data and distributing it to interested professionals can be significantly reduced. E-mail allows rapid visual communication between individuals or disseminating information to a number of people with the stroke of a single key.

Managed care companies are likely to make the Internet a means for connecting their provider networks. Precertifications, treatment reviews, and downloading new procedures or other news are potential uses. In general, the technology model is very attractive to MCCs because it is easier to collect and report information. The start-up costs are expensive and some therapists are technophobes. Yes, there is much to learn. But some of this will become a part of all our practices anyway; it's more a question of how far you want to go with it. This is where some of the younger clinicians who have grown up with computers may have an advantage over their more experienced competitors. By developing a reputation for innovation, you may be able to get contracts for special services to other providers/agencies. One risk is that it may not be what most consumers are looking for, yet. But it can be a good specialty strategy.

INTEGRATION STRATEGIES

This has become *the* hot topic in the managed care literature. Vertically integrated systems are more complex business arrangements in which you become part of a larger health care delivery system, typically with a group of hospitals at the core. Large groups will develop special programs such as partial day care for particular populations. But it can also involve outsourcing opportunities, in which the primary care system decides to hire a group to provide a set of services that would be more costly to develop itself, such as assessment or aftercare for a psychiatric hospital, a treatment compliance program for a surgical aftercare unit at a general hospital, or delivering outpatient mental health services in an outlying area for a large managed care organization.

Solo practitioners can operate similarly on a smaller scale, for example, contracting to provide services for a guidance center, medical or educational facility, Employee Assistance Program (EAP), or government program (e.g., disability assessments). Contracting out services is cheaper for companies because they don't have to pay benefits. You will have to comply with the regulations of the contractor, and the fee may be lower, but the arrangement can provide some stable income, and there is always the potential for additional referrals through these contacts.

These are vertical integration strategies. An example of a horizontal integration strategy is a coalition of group practices in a small geographic area, sharing specialties, referrals, and marketing costs. This strategy often makes it easier to fill groups or other specialty programs. The coalition can also create a separate, independent corporation called a management services organization (MSO), which provides all the administrative functions for a clinical network and can be very useful in seeking service contracts to cover a large geographic area.

The risks here are the time and money required to create and operate this type of system. It's not for those committed to solo or small group practices.

MANAGED CARE STRATEGY

This strategy involves you, as an individual therapist, being on the panels of the primary MCCs in your area and having a majority of your referrals come from them. In many areas, this is difficult to do now because panels are closed. But unique products can still get you on the list, as can setting up a second (or primary) location in an underserved area nearby. This strategy can be integrated with one or more of the other strategies. But for many therapists, this is their primary focus (creating some tension within the field between pro- and anti-managed care therapists). The risk is being dependent on companies that are in constant transition and having no (at present) legal protection of your role as a provider for any of them. There are also complex ethical and risk management issues.

Most of the new books about independent practice focus on how to survive in a managed care environment. Poynter (1994) and C. Browning and B. Browning (1994) are two good resources for those interested in developing a strong relationship with managed care companies. It is the strategy of choice for those who believe that working for MCCs will be the primary form of making a living as a mental health professional in the future. It is also an excellent opportunity for new clinicians, who are often better trained in the short-term techniques preferred by MCCs and will not experience the lower fees as a loss in income.

THE ALTERNATIVE INCOME STRATEGY

This is another of the hot topics in the 1990s. Every article on private practice emphasizes that there are many other ways to generate income besides direct patient treatment. It is, in fact, not only an opportunity for protecting or increasing your income, but also a source for some challenging and stimulating ways to apply your clinical skills. This strategy really isn't very new; a significant percentage of all private practitioners (the estimates range from a third to a half or even more) are in practice only part-time. Historically, teaching, training, consulting, and research have been a part of the life of many, if not most, mental health providers. But now nonpatient income is being heavily promoted by each of the professional organizations in order to reduce the anxiety of their members. It is being backed up with a substantial increase in continuing education programs designed to train people to add the special skills necessary to make alternative income sources a more viable (and ethical) possibility. The main opportunities tend to fall into six categories (please note this is not an exhaustive list).

1. **Legal:** forensics, expert witness, custody evaluations, special programs for drunk drivers and family violence, *guardian ad litem* (which may include custody work but goes further to include additional child protective services), divorce and civil mediation.
2. **Corporate:** executive coaching, outplacement, management consultation, wellness seminars, career counseling, training, employee screening, work/family programs, EAP services.
3. **Schools:** in-service training, contract services for testing or counseling, consulting.
4. **Psychoeducation:** all forms of workshops, retreats, and groups on special topics that are not psychotherapy (though they may have therapeutic benefits). They are usually time-limited and for cash (no third-party reimbursement, although some MCCs or insurance companies might contract for workshops on health-promoting topics). There is virtually no end to the list of topics.
5. **Government:** disability evaluations (including worker's compensation), consultation to federally funded programs.
6. **Training/Supervision:** Teaching providers how to do any of the above (continuing education has become a booming business), which includes offering supervision to providers in a variety of specialties.

There are many, many opportunities to expand your sources of income. But the trap here is the simplistic notion that it is easy to develop any of these as a viable competency. Too many providers are already rushing prematurely into new areas of practice without adequate training or recognition of the need for ongoing supervision. Furthermore, many of these options are already crowded with providers. All the marketing concepts being described in this book apply to these services as well as to traditional clinical practice.

8

Tactics:
Product, Place, and Price

Among the seven elements of the service marketing model, four are the traditional targets of creating tactical changes in order to increase revenues and profits. These are:

1. Product
2. Place
3. Price
4. Promotion

This chapter will deal with the first three elements. Promotion will be covered in Chapters 9 and 10.

PRODUCT

Historically our "product" has been psychotherapy. It's amazing to think about how we sold so much of it without any real marketing or promotional planning. Simultaneously, it is sobering to realize how the vast majority of people who could potentially benefit from our services don't use them. That's probably a direct result of the fact that we didn't market our product all these years. We were lazy and naïve. Now, in these more turbulent and competitive times, we no longer have the luxury of selling something as vague as psychotherapy. We need to break this complex of multiple activities into smaller units that are more easily defined to end users, both in terms of what is done and, especially, what it will do for the consumer. The important concept to keep in mind is that what you are selling has two key components: First, as discussed in Chapter 4, you are selling a process; second, you are selling outcomes, that is, those benefits that you can ethically promise to patients as likely results from using your particular service. Thus, mental health service products need to be promoted with markers that enable patients to evaluate the quality of the service and reduce the perception of risk in buying something they cannot see.

At the same time, I would note that the experience of receiving mental health services is something that patients can often evaluate much more easily than medical services. Patients can identify when they are feeling less depressed, are fighting less with a spouse, are less afraid to talk with strangers, or are able to improve school or work performance. It is less clear when a physician talks to you about what is going on inside your body unless you experience a reduction in symptoms. Patients who have made gains from psychotherapy probably tend to feel more confident about being able to maintain those gains in the future, because they usually have learned techniques to cope with the problem. In medicine, patients are more frequently passive recipients of treatments that they cannot see or control. Thus, the successful promotion of a mental health practice is dependent upon the development of definable mental health products, but the success of these products is dependent upon the success of the process required to deliver the product.

The most important concept in this section on products is that the narrower the service — the more focused, targeted, or specific it is — the easier it is to promote.

Thus, offering improved self-esteem in children through a specialized treatment approach is definitely a step in the right direction. But it is even better to narrow the focus to enhancing self-esteem in children with learning disabilities, or children with a chronic medical problem, or children who are jealous of an older sibling. Such highly specific products become easy to market. "Do you have a sibling rivalry problem in your family?" Once the readers of the ad or brochure say yes, they are hooked into what you have to say and they feel that you are speaking directly to them. Then you can offer a specific clinical service for a younger sibling who expresses jealousy, feels life is not fair, and may have other difficulties with peers or in school. You offer a program designed to help children feel better about themselves with a brief explanation of what it consists of and why it helps. It should produce phone calls from the type of patients you want to see and with whom you are particularly effective.

As you can see, product and promotion are so tightly linked that I am getting a bit ahead of myself. But I hope that you are already beginning to think about how to repackage one or more of your services into well-defined products. Here's just a brief list of some ideas for products:

- How to deal with a threatening boss.
- Overcoming test anxiety.
- Parent training for newly separated fathers.
- Marital therapy following spouse's bypass surgery.
- How to deal with separation anxiety in 6-year-olds.
- Forming new relationships after your spouse leaves you.
- Managing anger at the office.
- Dealing with sleep disturbances in toddlers.
- Surviving an affair.
- Prenuptial programs to develop marital relationship skills.
- Conflict resolution skills (couples or parent-child).
- Pain management.
- Dealing with migraines.
- A group for gifted 8- to 9-year-old girls with social problems (now *that's* specific and should be easy to market).
- Preparation to become a step-family.
- Relaxation training.
- Couples about to have their first child.

- Adjustment to cosmetic surgery.
- Performance enhancement.
- Post-surgery compliance.
- Families with a diabetic adolescent.
- Facing retirement.
- Coping with an aging parent.
- Parenting hyperactive children.

That should get your own creative juices flowing!

Your best service product is most likely something you already do. It may be only an occasional case, but during your internal assessment it's important to identify a patient population with whom you really enjoy working or a type of problem with which you are especially successful. In putting the product together into a package that can be promoted, don't be limited to traditional, weekly 50-minute sessions. Some of these products are better promoted as groups, and some would work better in 2-hour blocks on alternate weeks. It is best if many of them can have some time definition. One of the biggest patient resistances to psychotherapy is the fear of interminable length; another is the fear that, if therapy uncovers things patients may not be aware of, it will make them feel worse (which *can* happen and must be discussed with patients as one of the risks of psychotherapy). Time frames and focused treatment will help address both of these issues.

The key with time-limited products is to explain the goals up front but also to introduce the idea that continuing beyond that time period will be an option if the patient so desires. In my marital program, though it is advertised as a 12-session process, I explain that factors such as especially complex histories, patients who are detailed narrators, or current crises that require a time-out from the routine could extend the process by a few sessions. I explain that at the end of the 12 to 14 sessions, the couple will have a very clear sense of what their marital issues are, will have received some strategies for change, and may find that they don't need any further services. This happens about half the time. Other times, a couple may continue, on a weekly or less-frequent basis, because they want to continue to get help with their problems. Obviously the likelihood of this is higher when the presenting problem is more serious in either chronicity or intensity. In fact, if the couple is in open "warfare," I don't recommend the Marital Enhancement Therapy (MET) approach but offer a more solution-focused approach until the situation has improved. I also explain that in about 20% of couples, the ultimate decision is to get a divorce. This is scary but important to talk about. I find that in those cases the therapy usually results in a significantly less-acrimonious divorce.

Two important points emerge from this discussion. One is the importance of informed consent. Patients need to know what they are buying. Second, for those who are not committed to a practice of short-term therapy (that includes me; I much prefer the concept, which I believe I first heard at a seminar with Simon Budman, of time-sensitive therapy), it is important to have at least one or two time-sensitive products to be competitive in the current marketplace.

I hope that you are now comfortable with the concept of service products and how this can help you develop a mental health practice. As I have emphasized before, marketing skills benefit everyone. In developing products, you focus on your interests and clinical skills and consider ways to maximize your effectiveness. In turn, patients are probably more likely to benefit from such well-planned services (sorry, I have no data to back that up). Finally, specific products, with their promotional potential, are likely to draw more people to utilize your services. Maximizing quality and reaching more people who need mental health services are two of our most important ethical responsibilities.

PLACE

The location of your office is a critical part of your business. Its accessibility influences who can see you (e.g., Do they need a car? Do they have to climb stairs?). In addition, the design and furnishing of the office and waiting room influences how patients experience your services as well as their perception of you as a professional. This doesn't mean top-dollar fancy. It means creating an ambience and comfort that fits the image you are trying to project and has the patients' needs in mind. Is there adequate signage to make it easy to find you (some therapists provide maps or preprinted directions)? Is the waiting room comfortable, pleasant, and adequately lighted? Does it contain up-to-date, varied magazines and a play area for children? These may not be the critical issues for the majority of your patients, but they can be determining factors for some (which you'll never know about without collecting feedback) and simply a positive influence for others.

I keep copies of my columns in a notebook in my waiting room. Patients find it helpful and, especially for new patients, it solidifies their confidence in me. We also place bulletin boards on the walls and cover them with announcements of special programs, public relations announcements about people in the practice, newspaper articles on relevant topics, and even cartoons that provide a touch of humor about issues we work on. On the wall are holders for brochures — our own as well as those from national organizations — and materials about specific clinical problems. Many adult patients have accurately self-diagnosed ADD because of information they've read while waiting for an appointment.

Where you put your office is a variable you can change to possibly generate more referrals or reach a particular population you want to serve. If you want to get on a panel, open a satellite office in an underserved community. If you want more child referrals, open an office in a town that contains one of the fastest growing communities of young families. This often takes you further away from the major metropolitan area where you may currently practice. But the potential could be enormous. There is the option of having more than one location and reducing costs by splitting the space with an associate, each using the office half the time. Other specialized locations with specific benefits include an industrial park or a downtown financial district. This makes it easier to target the businesses in the areas and offers patients the option of scheduling appointments during the workday. For many it is much easier to walk 5 minutes to an office for an appointment which is built into a work schedule than to try driving somewhere before or after a day of work. You can take this a step further for busy executives by offering a version of home visits — come to *their* office! Obviously they would have to be comfortable with the possibility that others will know what is going on, but this is definitely not an issue for some when time is much more of a factor.

Another excellent location is in a group medical practice. This can result not only in typical referrals but also in opportunities for specialized services based on specific medical problem populations. And there is still the original office location — your home. The overhead is very low, and modern technology can link you to whatever resources you need. It can even be a selling point, with the greater emphasis on privacy and confidentiality as well as ambience. The key point is that location is something that should be carefully considered as an important part of the marketing of your practice. Avoid location by default; choose location to fit your goals.

PRICE

Pricing is a sensitive and complex issue, because mental health, unlike medical services, is a marketplace filled with different professionals offering essentially the same services for different fees. It is confusing to consumers and is part of the turf wars that divide our field and weaken our efforts to gain acceptance by the public, the corporate world, and the legislative process. It is also one of the central issues in the managed care debate, for fees have been arbitrarily set well below usual and customary levels. In addition, MCCs can reduce fees whenever they need to meet new financial goals for their contracts. The key point is that the more exposure one has to managed care, the less control one has over the price of one's services.

Nevertheless, fees remain a factor in a marketing plan. If you are a solo practitioner operating out of your own home with a very low overhead, it is possible to charge a fee significantly lower than your competitors and still have a higher net profit. If you are a new practitioner, offering services at a cut-rate fee over the first few years of your practice is a way to get established, that is, to gain market share. Once you have established the quality of your services and built up an adequate demand, you can begin to steadily raise your fees until they are more in line with the competition. As described in the chapter on practice strategies, fees are (or should be) linked to your primary choice of strategy. Specialists and experts can charge more; low-cost, high-volume practitioners would be charging less. External factors also influence fees. The more affluent the community, or the higher the percentage of traditional indemnity insurance in your area, the higher your fee can be.

One of the increasing trends in our field is the policy of collecting fees at the session rather than billing at the end of the month. Many therapists offer a discount for doing this, because it improves cash flow and saves money. Insurance factors may limit this practice, because a number of companies require direct billing or limit out-of-pocket expense to a copayment. Another issue is whether your fees are fixed or flexible. You have to be very careful with flexible fees, as there are serious questions about the legalities. For example, you cannot bill the insurance company at your regular fee if you have charged the patient a reduced fee. Another question is the legality of reducing fees after insurance has run out. You *must* collect copayments. Flexible fees are easiest to use for uninsured patients, and may be used as exceptions for cases when insurance coverage has ended. Although the majority of therapists appear to have some flexibility in their fees, others insist on full-fee-only and prefer to offer stretched-out, monthly payment plans to make therapy affordable. This is particularly effective for therapists who specialize in short-term treatment. Another way to deal with this issue is to use credit cards. Although you pay a small fee for the service, it improves cash flow and enables patients with limited finances to work out their own payment process at their expense rather than yours.

A controversial price issue is offering free services, usually in the form of an initial consultation or a short-term, psychoeducational group. Some therapists feel this is unprofessional; others see it as a reasonable way to enable patients to shop for a therapist they like. The key is always to find a way to get people into your office and then allow the quality of your services to be the ultimate selling point. I do not offer free initial sessions. The explanation to those who ask why not is that an hour spent with me will produce beneficial feedback. Thus I am working and the patient is benefiting. That's the essential reason for me to be charging a fee, so I do. As for free groups, this is supposed to provide a source of individual patients, but my analysis of the examples I've read about is that when you add the cost of therapy time lost plus marketing expenses, the return isn't worth it.

Another fee manipulation is to charge less for hours that are harder to fill. However, my experience is that if you establish a demand for your services there is no need to do this. It's amazing how even very busy people manage to find an hour during the week when they really want to. But if you're having trouble filling hours, this may help.

In examining product, place, and price you have a significant number of ways to alter your current practice and increase your success.

9

Promotion:
Selling; Public Relations

There are four types of promotion: public relations (PR), advertising, sales promotions, and personal selling. Most of the relevant promotional activity for a private practitioner will fall into the first two categories, PR and advertising. Each is an essential and major component to an effective marketing plan. However, the two sales-related promotions do have a potential usefulness, even if limited. So I will start with a brief summary of sales promotions and personal selling and then move on to the main focus — public relations. Advertising will be covered in Chapter 10.

SELLING

Sales promotions are using special inducements designed to motivate people to immediately try sampling your services. This is a very commercial aspect of promotion and has not been used very much with outpatient mental health services. However, it has some potential. I mentioned earlier the question of giving free initial consultations and charging less for certain hours of the day. These are forms of sales promotions. If there are certain times of the year that are slow (e.g., summers), try offering special reduced fees for short-term interventions during the summer. Another idea would be to develop an arrangement with a corporation in your area; in exchange for the opportunity to leave promotional material on site (or to give a free workshop), employees would pay a reduced fee for your services. Again, these are not likely to appeal to the average therapist, but for some they can provide the extra edge needed to get established or expand the business.

Personal selling is a ridiculously underutilized aspect of most small practices. After all, we are in the relationship business.* Yet, we expend very little energy in developing face-to-face relationships with potential sources of referrals. Whether it's with a local physician, a guidance counselor, a community worker, an attorney, or an EAP or managed care staff person, we rarely call and ask to meet. Clinical readers can guess at the dynamics of this phenomenon. My point is that you are missing out on one of the best ways to develop referrals. Remember that people are busy and it's very competitive out there. So have a reason for them to meet with you. This brings us back to one of the most important concepts in this book: how to differentiate yourself from other therapists. You need to offer potential contacts something that is a bit special or different.

Sometimes, especially in smaller communities, it is not so essential to emphasize this uniqueness up front. People are often willing to meet you as long as there is some implied sense that you are simply a very competent clinician who can be of benefit to their clients. This, of course, is the other frequent theme on these pages: The cornerstone of any successful practice is quality of services.

Please remember that personal selling is not a one-shot deal. Relationships are not built in single meetings. Periodically re-

---

*Psychotherapy research increasingly points to one of the key factors in successful outcomes as getting patients to buy in to your way of explaining their problem. Pure and simple, it is the selling of yourself to your patients as a knowledgeable and competent professional that is essential to successful psychotherapy. So don't knock the role of selling in the business of psychotherapy.

turn, especially when you've added something new to your practice, or just to touch base once again and see if there is any way you can be of service to them. This latter point is a key in selling. First learn what the buyer is looking for: "What kinds of psychological problems impact on the people you deal with?" "How can I be of help to you in your work?" "What kind of feedback would you want from me if you make a referral?" Approach people with the idea that you are doing them a favor by offering help instead of thinking that you are trying to get something from them. Again, this requires you to believe that you have something special to offer: service products and a level of competence that makes you different from your competitors. Phone calls and/or thank-you notes are an important part of reinforcing this relationship. Holiday cards also help to keep your name in front of the key people who send you business. Holiday baskets, especially to the office staff — who are often the key people who direct referrals — are a particularly nice way to say thanks.

PUBLIC RELATIONS

The objective of PR is to make the public aware of you, what services you provide, and (very important in our business) the value of these services. Because you are not likely to be able to afford to hire a PR staff person, you will need to learn how to do this yourself. The concept is not difficult. A good start is to read Michael Levine's *Guerrilla P.R.* (1993). The book is fun to read because of all the anecdotes about celebrities, and, as the title suggests, it is oriented to the small businessperson.

Levine's concept is that the goal is not merely getting publicity but rather using media to establish a positive feeling toward you. In other words, it's about emotion. That certainly should give us an edge in how to do this right. Levine believes that media is the second strongest influence on people's lives, right behind family; that media creates "truths" in the minds of its audience. Some say psychotherapy does the same thing; that is, that we give people a way of understanding their lives in order to enable them to make changes in their behavior.

There is an additional special connection between PR and mental health: The person considered to be the founder of modern public relations was Edward Bernays, a nephew of Freud!

Good PR is simply using creative thinking toward a goal of shaping your image and then getting that image into the public's awareness. It usually involves very minimal costs, so it is especially helpful for therapists with very limited budgets. You need to create a strong image of what you do, who it helps, and what it does for them. If you can accomplish those three goals, then you have a powerful PR campaign.

To be a success at "Guerrilla P.R." (GPR), "you must retain a healthy and positive sense of self-importance" (Levine, 1993, p. 22). In running my workshops, I found this to be one of the most difficult issues for mental health professionals. When I asked for a show of hands as to who thought they were a competent therapist, the whole room waved at me. When I asked how many believed they were very important in the lives of their patients, once again, the air was filled with raised arms. But when I asked how many would walk outside this room and tell other people how competent they were and how important their work could be to people's lives, very few participants raised a hand. Why is it that we are so reluctant to promote ourselves, in a professional manner, to people outside our profession? Workshop participants nearly always answer that they have been taught that to do so is *not* professional. But you can do PR in a very professional manner.

I think there is another issue imbedded here, especially for the solo practitioner. You are used to operating outside of public scrutiny. Patients are sent to you through personal referral sources, and your work is largely confidential. Until now, outcomes have consisted only of your personal sense of how often you help your patients. To go public is to make yourself visible to a much larger audience who may question your competence and may even ask for some proof of competence. It tests our belief in ourselves. Alone, in the confines of our office, where we have the upper hand as "the professional," we feel safer in promoting our sense of knowledge and competence. To promote this sense of competence in more public ways through workshops, written articles, brochures, and other forms of PR is to invite public scrutiny. It tests your true sense of confidence in what you do.

GPR philosophy is based on the notion that while you appear to be trying to appeal to the masses, you are actually trying to persuade individuals, one at a time, to take action and seek out your services. It's important to think of it in these terms. When you give a talk, you don't expect the entire group of 25 to 30 people to call you the next day to set up an appointment. In fact, it may be weeks, months, or even years later when people who have listened to your presentation have the need and think of you as the person to fill that need. And that will be true only for a very few of the people who heard you that night. So your goal is to make a strong impression on a few individuals and repeat that over and over. Those people who walk away with a particularly positive impression of you are not simply potential patients but are now ambassadors of promotion of your services. It is not unusual for a new patient to identify his or her source of referral as someone who once heard me speak.

To be successful at GPR you must look at the strengths and weaknesses you identified in your internal analysis. Are you a good speaker, writer, or a cold caller (calling on people you've never met)? Are you artistic, especially knowledgeable about certain topics, good at handling questions from an audience, able to talk about mental health issues in everyday language, and willing to invest money and time in promoting yourself? Do you have products that differentiate your practice from the competition? Do you know who comprises your target audience, and do you have a way to convey how your services will benefit them?

In whatever format you try to reach people, the key is for it to feel very personal to your audience. You need stories — everybody loves stories — that strike a personal chord in the listener/reader. I love hearing from new callers that my ad/brochure/presentation/article made them feel as if I were talking about their life; as if I already knew about their problem. They feel a connection to me that starts therapy on a very positive note, a very different cathexis than patients simply referred by someone.

Much of Levine's book deals with developing a relationship with the media. This is his specialty as the foremost PR consultant to the stars. Levine believes that print media is most effective because the printed word makes the most lasting impression in people's minds. He emphasizes magazines over newspapers, but that is a very difficult medium for most of us to crack. He gives us some insights into the world of journalists, whom he describes as always skeptical but also always in need of a good story. I was surprised to read that most stories are brought to journalists, because they don't have time to go out and find enough stories to constantly fill their pages.

You are not a PR professional, but what you may lack in skills is counterbalanced by your sincerity. You are very invested in what you are promoting; you truly believe in its value. This can help get you past the skepticism of journalists who are used to contrived stories that have no intrinsic value but are merely efforts to get someone's name in print. If you are going to attempt to approach a media person, Levine emphasizes that you must know your subject thoroughly (the competence issue), have an interesting story to tell (the media operates on the principal that the public is always bored with what is and to get their attention you need something new, preferably controversial), and be familiar with the specific media person or source that you have approached: You should have read the paper or the magazine, or watched/listened to the show a number of times before reaching out. Also, be persistent. You may get turned down many times before coming up with the right idea at the right time.

Let me give you a few personal examples. *Example #1:* Over a year ago I realized that our group practice (which started with just two people in 1974) was approaching its 20th anniversary, and I thought that might make for an interesting article in our local paper. I spoke to the editor of the paper, who expressed interest, especially because we offered to write a draft (local papers have very small staffs). One of our therapists then wrote a story that reflected on changes in society and mental health over the past two decades with a sprinkling of quotes from various group members. (Note: journalists love quotes!) After a few revisions, we presented the story to the editor, who promised he would have one of his writers talk to me and make some revisions and then publish it. We were very excited, but many months went by and nothing happened. I periodically asked, and was always told they would get around to it.

Finally, early in 1995, he assigned someone to the story and it was published, using my picture as the founder of the practice. Many people in town commented on the article. They knew many of us individually but didn't realize we were associated, especially for so long (at that time there were 14 therapists), and it also gave us a chance to educate the public just a little bit about the benefits of mental health services.

I do not know of a specific referral that was generated by the article. But the PR value was enormous. It generated a significant increase in awareness of us in the community, and I'm certain that when other forms of promotion took place, the cumulative effect did lead to referrals (which have increased dramatically over the past 2 years in response to the group ad we ran in the local paper). We also posted the article on the bulletin board in our waiting rooms. Because most of our patients come from towns where the article did not appear, it gave them a chance to read about us and added to their confidence in us.

Example #2: Over the past few years there has been a growth in so-called "safety classes." These are educational programs targeting preschool and early elementary grade children with the objective of teaching them how not to become victims of child sexual abuse or what to do if they are victimized. As a child and family specialist, I strongly disagreed with these classes for a number of reasons. During 1994, two of the articles that I read on this subject distressed me to the point of taking action. I wrote a letter to the editor of the *Journal of Child Sexual Abuse* (JCSA) and one to the publisher of a local, and very popular, publication called *The Boston Parents' Paper* (TBPP). Neither was written with the intent of getting published; the *Journal* didn't have a "Letters" section, and my letter was far too long for the Boston paper; it was merely meant to be educational. Yet both got printed! JCSA decided to start a "Letters" section. Of course, as with most journals, a year passed before the letter actually appeared in print. Meanwhile, the publisher of TBPP felt my comments would be very informative to her readers, so it was published immediately.

About a year later I received a call from a local TV news reporter who wanted to do a two-part piece on safety classes. She had read my *Parents' Paper* article and filed it for future reference. After a telephone discussion which resulted in my sending her some articles to read, I was called again (months later) and suddenly she appeared in my office with a cameraman for a 20-minute interview. Of course, only about a minute of it appeared over the two nights, but thousands of people got a brief introduction to me. The TV station liked me and took information about what other topics I could speak on. Early in 1997, I was again interviewed (this time in my home) on a controversial court case. This time a longer segment was shown several times in the course of the weekend. Maybe somebody out there will now recognize my name more readily and end up choosing to call me instead of somebody else.

The important point to remember about PR (and other promotional tactics) is that if you keep getting your name out there, good things will happen, sometimes in unexpected ways. This was partly an example of someone coming to me.

Levine explains in detail how to approach the media. Start by developing a mailing list — primarily a local list of the editors, TV and radio hosts, and writers who target your areas of expertise. However, even though it may seem like a remote possibility to you, a national list may also produce a surprising opportunity. Your national professional organization may even have a media division that can be very helpful in this regard. And your state organization may have a speaker's bureau and/or a media resource list. (If they don't, push them to create one.)

The key, as always in promotion for the solo practitioner, is to have a specialty. The objective is to get on someone's list so when they need an opinion in that area of specialization, they might give you a call. Once you have developed your mailing list, Levine recommends putting together a "press kit." This includes a letter of introduction, a brief bio, a good black-and-white photo, and copies of articles and press clippings. The bio should be a statement no longer than two paragraphs that clearly defines your areas of expertise, experience in media (if any), and a very brief statement of professional credentials. You may also enclose a CV (curriculum vitae) if it solidifies your expertise. You may send this kit to the people on your mailing list and simply ask them to keep you on their list as a potential resource for a story/show in your specialty area. Another approach, for the print media, is to send the kit with a cover letter in which you briefly outline an article that you have written which you believe has market value and ask if they would be interested. Follow up the mailing with a phone call. Don't wait for them to call you. Keep in mind that they are only going to be interested in printing something that has some "pop" to it, something that will catch the reader's attention. For a local paper, the sizzle may be less important than an interesting local theme. As with all other aspects of marketing, you must be persistent and recognize that you are making a long-term investment. The first few opportunities are usually the hardest to come by, but once you are able to list some radio/TV appearances or enclose some newspaper or magazine articles, you will be taken more seriously and your list will grow steadily.

Here is an annotated list of 16 promotional tactics. Examine the list and consider which of these best fits your style, skills, and budget. The more you can commit to, the easier it will be to achieve the PR goal of establishing a positive emotional awareness of you in the minds of your targeted population, increasing the likelihood of being contacted for your services.

LOGO

It can be helpful if all of your printed material displays a logo that conveys an image of you and/or your services. Though it is not essential, consistent use of a logo assists people in remembering who you are. There are public-domain software programs that offer many logos to choose from. A graphic designer can show this to you or help you design a unique one. Obviously the former is much cheaper.

STATIONERY

Put some thought into your selection of stationery. It is one of the most frequently used items that conveys an image of you. It should contain your logo, if you have one. It should list your associates if you are part of a small group. It might identify your affiliation with a major educational or medical institution. It can also include a line at the bottom that helps to establish in the minds of readers something special about you. In other words, your stationery can be a form of advertising/promotion — not just a piece of paper to write on. For example, my tag line, used on all advertising and promotional materials, is "Helping Children, Families, Couples, and Adults Since 1968." This tag line emphasizes the important points about my practice: my helpfulness, the populations I work with, and my extensive experience. It is consistent with the idea that everything I do and everything about my practice is an opportunity to promote both information about and an image of who I am.

BUSINESS CARD

The same concepts apply. I am currently using a soft-cream-colored, textured stationery stock with matching card. The card also includes the group logo and the promotional line described above. My card doubles as an appointment card on the back. Some people prefer to separate these functions. The main point is to remind you that you hand out your card to a wide variety of people. Therefore, it should be distinctive and provide more than just the basic information. It is an opportunity, albeit a brief one, to tell the recipient something important about who you are and what you do. Take advantage of it. Business cards are very inexpensive promotional items.

CURRICULUM VITAE (CV)

A holdover from our academic backgrounds, CVs are traditionally used instead of resumés. I recommend that if you are going to consider yourself a businessperson, use a modified form of the traditional CV that incorporates an essential component of a good resumé. The first page is designed to emphasize what makes you unique; to highlight your strengths, specialties, and accomplishments. Educational history is pushed back, and job history must emphasize special achievements. If you are using this to impress media people, then media experiences need a prominent place. In other words, professional credentials are less important than telling people what you do and conveying a sense of how well you do it.

COMMUNITY INVOLVEMENT, NONPROFESSIONAL

An important way to become known is to become active in some religious or civic group, making sure to take opportunities to let people know what you do. It is not only a rewarding expenditure of time, but it achieves a number of promotional goals such as the image of your being a giving and caring person, and your ability to get things done. It also provides opportunities to meet people who may be potential referral sources or connections to media opportunities.

One frequently overlooked option is to join the local business association — this means thinking of yourself as a businessperson. Sometimes this provides an opportunity to give a presentation or to open up possibilities of doing work in the business community. None of this is meant to diminish true civic commitment or turn it into a business activity — I just completed 2 years as president of a community agency; because it involved many, many hours, this commitment had to come from the heart. But as people came to know what I did for a living (and people are fascinated with our field), it ultimately led to some increased business opportunities. I didn't push that aspect, but I was always aware of it. Sometimes I was specifically tapped, for example, talking to phys-ed staff on how to work with hyperactive children, or to preschool teachers on dealing with aggressive behavior in the classroom. Being a psychologist is a part of who I am. I never forget it and I try to make it a value-added aspect of anything I can do for the community.

COMMUNITY INVOLVEMENT, PROFESSIONAL

Giving talks, especially free ones for a variety of community groups, is one of the best ways to generate referrals. If you are not comfortable with public speaking, get some training. You have a wealth of knowledge about topics people love to listen to and ask questions about. If you have developed specialties, as I keep emphasizing, then you will be repeatedly asked to speak on those topics. The more you become known, the possibility increases that organizations with a speakers' budget will contact you; this can become an additional source of income. One plus is that the more you speak, the less preparation time is required. You'll have your notes in a folder and the concepts will flow easily. Some fine-tuning to fit the specific audience and you'll be a hit. To get things rolling, you may need to contact agencies and groups to tell them about yourself and the topics you can speak about. Look at the community listings in your local paper to find out who is inviting speakers.

Use presentations as an opportunity to promote yourself in a tangible way. I always prepare packets and place one on every seat based on the estimated number of attendees. In each packet I include my own brochure, the group practice brochure, my business card, copies of some relevant articles I've written (if you don't have that, you can substitute an outline of the presentation and/or a summary of your key points, a list of recommended readings, or a copy of an article written by someone else that supports your ideas), and a few pieces of blank paper for taking notes. These packets are rarely left behind, and I know from experience that the materials get shared with others. I always bring extras because people often ask to take materials to a friend who couldn't make it.

As another example of how promotional activities grow into new opportunities, it is not unusual to have someone in the audience come up and ask you to speak for another organization that he or she is also involved with.

Another form of professional community involvement is to volunteer time in a community agency where your skills are needed. Free consultation or service time creates a positive image and will likely lead to referrals (ethically they can't be directly related to your consultations), because people will get to know your skills and send you friends and others who could benefit from your services.

Volunteering to teach a psychology class at your local high school is a fun way to gain some exposure. The teachers are often eager to have a professional come in and talk about specialty topics or just explain more about what mental health professionals do. Also, most high schools have career days, and it is rewarding to work with teens eager to learn about your profession. In the meantime, you have gained exposure to high school staff and directly to many teens, all of which can be helpful if you treat adolescents.

Most public schools run adult education programs. Although the pay is usually minimal, it is excellent exposure to teach a course, especially on popular lay topics such as stress management, procrastination, time management, parenting, and marital communication. The nice part of this promotional strategy is that all the advertising is done for you and your name will end up in every house in town! Schools also run in-service training programs. Providing workshops to staff can be an excellent way to reach potential referral sources.

Another fruitful way to build helpful community relationships is to present at a community hospital Grand Rounds. Being on staff is also a good way to connect to the local medical community.

In your area there will be local chapters of many health-related organizations. Some are specific to mental health issues (e.g., ADD, major psychiatric illnesses, Obsessive Compulsive Disorder [OCD]), others to medical problems where your input would be well received (e.g., cancer, multiple sclerosis, cerebral palsy). Also, there will be area planning boards in most states that oversee public programs in mental health and mental retardation. Joining them not only offers exposure to influential community people and the opportunity to influence the delivery of services, but sometimes it makes you aware of opportunities to develop new programs through state and federal grants.

SPECIAL COMMUNITY PROMOTIONS

With the arrival of nationally sponsored "recognition" days for various mental health problems, there is an excellent opportunity to work with the local health care community. This often leads to direct referrals. Some examples are: "National Depression Screening Day," "National Anxiety Screening Day," and "National Eating Disorders Screening Day." There will probably be more by the time you are reading this! Often these programs are run in collaboration with community hospitals, and there is an opportunity for you to be involved.

Similar community events are town health fairs, a wonderful opportunity to educate people about mental health. You can obtain brochures on a variety of mental health topics from professional organizations plus distribute your own materials. It is not only excellent exposure, but it also helps increase people's knowledge about mental health problems and services. Colleges frequently sponsor health fairs for their students; working with this population is an excellent opportunity for exposure.

Other civic events that you normally may not pay attention to may offer excellent opportunities to become known among town business leaders. Typically these are fund-raisers. Our local business association sponsors an annual spelling bee. We now send a team each year; it adds to our local recognition and reinforces a view that we care about our community, which is wonderful small-town PR.

A similar local PR project that we started this year is to offer a small scholarship ($200) to a graduating high school senior who is committed to a career in mental health. The local newspaper printed a photograph and accompanying story when we awarded the check to the deserving student.

Remember that all this is about making people aware of who you are and what you do. Many of these ideas are fun and bring with them the added satisfaction of contributing to community welfare. Even as a solo practitioner, you can pick doable projects; sometimes, a few independent therapists can share a project.

PROFESSIONAL ORGANIZATION INVOLVEMENT

This is something you should be doing no matter what your practice needs are. In these challenging times, we need a lot of grass-roots involvement. The key is to never lose sight of how this can be of help to your goal of building a practice. The primary means of accomplishing this in a professional organization is taking advantage of the fact that you have a chance to inform many colleagues of your areas of specialization and to demonstrate that you are a caring and competent person in the work you do within the organization. You may write for publications, chair a committee on one of your specialties, or give workshops at annual meetings (the latter two help to establish your role as an expert outside the organization and may result in colleagues referring cases that they do not treat). You may also enjoy talking to politicians, corporate executives, or insurance executives. This, too, can lead to new opportunities.

MEDIA INTERVIEWS

This results, of course, when a media professional has responded to your press kit about your areas of expertise and your willingness (and ability) to provide some good copy. One general rule about interviews is never give the interview on the initial phone call. Clarify what the person is looking for, explain you need to finish something (e.g., a patient is waiting), and arrange a specific time to return the call. The reason for the delay is to organize your thoughts. What are the key points you want to make? Can you provide some good examples, that is, the stories that everybody wants to hear? Make a few notes and then call the interviewer back as soon as possible. Most of my calls come from the local newspapers. Only recently have I begun to get into some of the city papers and area TV. But local papers are your bread and butter because they are more likely to produce referrals.

PROFESSIONAL PUBLICATIONS

Although the average potential patient is not interested in reading your latest journal article or reviewing your list of citations, professional publications are an important part of establishing yourself as an expert and can be woven gently into promotional materials. It can be especially helpful in getting recognized by journalists. It can also increase recognition of your special expertise by colleagues and thus lead to referrals.

PRESS RELEASES

This is often the heart of the job of a PR specialist. It's that wonderful free exposure of your name in the media. For solo or small group practices, you should develop a list of which local newspapers will print news about talks, awards, and publications. Ask for the format for delivering the information to them. Create a form and regularly send it out to your sources. If you are an active professional, hardly a month will go by that you can't put some announcement in the local paper. This is easier to do if you have a secretary to take care of it as a routine process. Even solo practitioners should have a part-time secretary to handle tasks such as these.

Remember, the goal is to maximize the exposure that keeps putting you in the minds of the public, so when they are in need of mental health services, your name will seem familiar to them and they will be more likely to call you. Also, any form of PR has the potential to lead to requests for other promotional opportunities. Thus, an announcement that you have given a presentation may lead someone to call and ask if you would give that presentation to their organization.

TRAINING OF PROFESSIONALS

This has been mentioned as an alternative source of income, but it is also another method of self-promotion. If you have special skills that qualify you to train other mental health professionals, it is also likely that they will think of you at times as a person to refer to, particularly in the specialty area that you are supervising.

LAY PUBLICATIONS

This is probably one of the most effective promotional techniques, but it requires writing skill and a significant commitment to getting published. The marketplace is already flooded with a mental health columnist in most major magazines and newspapers, and bookshelves are packed with health care titles. The easiest entry point, as always, is local. Look for community or area newspapers or local magazines that might be targeted for a regular feature or an occasional article. Be persistent. It took a few years of trying before I found an outlet for my column on parenting, but now it appears in seven towns. Also, it took years before it became a routine source of new referrals.

Be creative when it comes to exploring magazines or specialty publications. The hot focus in magazines is narrow populations; you may be able to create a psychological column with a twist for that particular specialty. Also, many large organizations publish regular newsletters where there might be an opportunity for a good column. Your state bar association or medical society, state chapters for learning disability associations, medical specialty organizations, area business publications, or other specialty publications are all potential outlets for your insights and advice. For example, I learned about a company that produces promotional quarterlies for certain businesses. One such local business using it is called "Parents-in-a-Pinch," which provides child care for sick children. Their quarterly publication, designed to promote their service among dual-income families and single parents, is distributed at corporations. I was approached to place an ad and ended up working out a deal that would include one of my columns in each issue. Great exposure!

Use the *Writer's Market* annual as a guide (see References list at the end of this book) in attempting to become published in lay venues. It is an excellent resource.

Writing a book is a dream for many of us, but only a tiny percentage make it to the stores. But don't be put off by this harsh reality. If you can write and can come up with a creative, unique way to say something to the public, then go for it. There are courses to help navigate these challenging waters.

Even if sales are small (and don't expect to get rich even if sales are big), just being an author is great for PR when it comes to getting speaking engagements and promoting yourself as an expert.

MAILINGS

This should be an essential component of any marketing plan for a small practice. The key is deciding who to mail to and what to send them. There is a multitude of choices. You must build a plan that is consistent with your goals and complements other strategies. The possibilities include targeting current referral sources, potential referral sources, former patients, current patients, and potential patients. My preference is for semiannual mailings to actual and potential referral sources that describe services offered, including any special new programs, or introducing a new member of the group. The mailings can include brochures and/or newsletters (which I will discuss in the chapter on advertising) or can simply be letters. With a computer and a mailing program plus a laser printer, you can produce a quality mailing that can be either general or targeted. Mailing software allows you to easily organize your list by several criteria, so you could send a mailing just to physicians or guidance counselors — and even that can be refined to a specific geographic area via zip codes. This fits with themes of keeping your name in front of people, with themes of the need for repetition, and with emphasis on how you are different from other therapists in at least one significant way. In addition to regular mailings, there are specialty mailings for a new service such as a mailing to guidance counselors to announce a new program for ADHD, or to attorneys for a new divorce support program.

A few key points for successful mailings: Always use quality stationery. If you can, address by hand, because those letters are more likely to be opened. Your first line has to offer a compelling reason for the reader to want to read on — it must promise something of strong interest or need to the reader. Mailings are especially effective if a follow-up phone call is promised and made. That usually requires mailings to be small in volume — very targeted — which is consistent with the time and money of a solo practitioner. Don't get discouraged. It may take a few years of regular mailings before you see the payoff. Remember, many start the process, but few continue it. Your persistence, the cornerstone of an effective marketing campaign, will establish a sense of stability and permanence in your readers that will gradually persuade some of them to build a relationship with you.

Mailings to patients, current or former, should be done only if signed consent has been obtained, to respect privacy and the confidentiality of the treatment relationship. Keeping patients aware of new services can be an excellent source of new referrals. Mailings to former patients sometimes serve to stimulate their return for some extra help. I prefer to communicate with current patients via waiting-room bulletin boards or enclosures in monthly billing statements. I haven't used mailings to former patients, but others have reported it to be useful.

More expensive direct mailing programs can involve buying mailing lists targeted in some particular way to fit your practice. The return is small, however, for this type of mailing, so the financial return probably doesn't justify the cost. However, you can create your own specialized mailing lists out of your local town hall. Street listings usually contain information on the ages and occupations of residents. So if you want to reach parents of school-age children or seniors or affluent families (potential cash customers), you could generate your own specialized mailing list.

RADIO

This has also become a very competitive area for promotion. Many cities have call-in shows featuring mental health specialists. However, you may be able to sell yourself to a local station. This obviously takes a certain personality and is best done by those who know their topic and understand the ethics of giving over-the-air advice. When done properly, radio shows not only generate business but also serve as a positive source of education about mental health issues and services. It's always easier to crack a field like this if you have established yourself with the media, but often, like the rest of life, it's simply a matter of knowing someone who is in a position to give you a chance to demonstrate your skill. Don't be afraid to ask friends who might have contacts in the business.

TV

TV exposure usually means one of two activities — being a guest (or regular) expert on a local show (morning shows, talk shows, news shows) or creating your own local cable show. The former is covered under earlier comments about developing press kits and reaching out to local media specialists in mental health issues. As always, it helps if you have been able to establish yourself as an expert in some area. You may tire of my emphasis on the need to develop a specialty (or two), but the name of the game is to differentiate yourself from thousands of other mental health professionals.

One of my favorite recommendations is to use local cablevision. These stations are required to do local programming and are often starving for good (and inexpensive) material. Mental health topics are always popular, and if you can come up with a good idea for an interesting show, there's a good chance you will get an opportunity to try it. Although some question the size and nature of the audience for local cable shows, you can also help the station promote it in the local newspaper and build an audience. Frequently, one cablevision system owns the stations in many towns in your area, and a good show will be shown in neighboring communities. A couple of years ago our group agreed to offer a series of free lectures on parenting in collaboration with the town's Department of Public Health. It was done at the local hospital and our cable station agreed to tape and televise each of the lectures. It was a great deal for everyone.

Brochures and newsletters could be considered as forms of PR, but because of the special costs and design involved, I believe they are more akin to advertising, so they will be covered in the next chapter.

10

Promotion: Advertising

Historically, advertising has been avoided by health care providers. In fact, until just a few years ago, it was considered unethical for psychologists to advertise. But the Federal Trade Commission required the American Psychological Association to change the rules, establishing what was obvious to many: We are in business and we can't be prohibited from informing the public about our services. For many health care providers, however, advertising is still thought to be unprofessional, associated with only the most negative aspects of commercialism. Also, some marketing consultants say that advertising is not effective in the managed care marketplace because so many people are limited in their choice of providers. I disagree. I simply set my goals for new referrals one-third higher to account for possible out-of-panel rejections. In addition, many of these people (about 15%) end up paying out of pocket, which is one of my goals. Also, the insurance market may change due to point-of-service contracts or any-willing-provider legislation or some new idea that hasn't been thought of yet. I intend to be a survivor, and advertising is one of the key ways to make people aware of who I am and what I can do for them.

Advertising can be done in a quality, professional manner and serves to inform people about the value of mental health services while identifying you as someone who can help. Sturdivant's (1990) research indicated that consumers have positive reactions to mental health advertising. So it's our issue, not theirs. We need to stop projecting our misgivings onto the public. Advertising helps people make choices. In the current, highly competitive marketplace, I consider it one of our most effective tools. It is clearly one of the most time-proven techniques for increasing business. I like to advertise because my time is in shorter supply than my money (within reason, of course), and because ads have generated a steady supply of referrals plus calls from people looking for speakers, workshop leaders, and consultants (and people wanting you to advertise in their publications!).

Mental health advertising must follow guidelines established by our various national organizations. Professional standards require factual, nondeceptive ads that inform consumers and do not manipulate emotions. We must be very careful to promise only what can be delivered. Ads that work best usually convey a sense of warmth, as if you were talking directly to the readers about their specific concerns. Don't promote your credentials. Consumers are interested in the benefits of your services, not your degrees. As Levinson (1990) puts it, women do not buy shampoo, they buy beautiful, clean, or manageable hair.

Your advertising plan should be consistent with your practice goals and with the strategies you are using to achieve those goals. Everything should fit together. This includes emphasis on the importance of developing specialties. It is much easier to design ads for specialty services than for generic therapies. As always, you must keep in mind that you are investing in your practice with a long-term view. It usually takes at least 6 months before any promotional or marketing efforts begin to show results. On the other hand, when it does start to pay dividends, if you keep working at it, the gains tend to become cumulative and increasingly powerful.

WHERE TO ADVERTISE

The key is being able to be as efficient as possible with your advertising dollars. Efficiency refers to reaching the audience that is most likely to contain the maximum number of people who will want and are able to purchase your services. This is referred to as targeting. Local weekly newspapers and specialty publications probably give you the best return for each dollar spent. Big city dailies are very costly, as are magazines, radio, and TV. Plus they reach a broad audience, most of whom are unlikely to come to your location. There are exceptions, such as promoting a workshop, when you may want the one-shot, expensive approach. But the best advertising is repetitious. The ad needs to be seen over and over, promoting an increased sense of familiarity as well as being there at the particular moment when the need is also present. For this reason, I regularly turn down requests to buy space in ad books (unless you are doing so strictly to make a donation to the organization) because those one-shot listings do not produce business. On our limited budgets, we need to find the lower cost venues that give us the best return.

One commonly overlooked resource is organization newsletters: local bar association, medical society, associations for the learning disabled or mentally ill, and special community agencies. For example, I run a very inexpensive ad in a newsletter for a local parent support organization which has about 300 to 400 members, primarily parents of very young children. It not only produces an occasional referral but it is introducing me to these parents and may result in more referrals as their children get older. I have combined this with giving some parenting workshops and publishing a few parenting articles in the newsletter. The combination has resulted in a significant number of referrals. (I differentiate the source of the referral, so I know who called just from the ad as opposed to having heard me speak and/or read an article.) This underscores one of the key themes of *Guerrilla Marketing Weapons* (Levinson, 1990) and of this book — use as many of the promotional tactics as you can as consistently as possible, because it is the combination of ways to get your name out there and keep it out there that will generate referrals.

For those who practice in big cities, there are many neighborhood publications or weekly newspapers that serve parts of the city. There are also local magazines that can be very effective if the readers are particularly well suited for your specialty services. Most publications have detailed descriptions of their readers, and you should review that before placing an ad to make sure you are reaching the right audience and that the circulation numbers fit the costs. In some cases, such as *The Boston Parents' Paper,* which reaches over 100,000 families in my area, the decision is a no-brainer. This has been the location of my most effective advertising. When I decided to develop marital therapy as one of my major "products," I began running an ad in this paper. It took until the second year (and a few design changes) before it started generating referrals. By the fourth year, it was producing an average of three calls and 1.5 new referrals a month. Also, in keeping with the multiple-tactic approach, I finally convinced the editor to publish a couple of articles (usually their writers are parents who freelance), and each one resulted in additional calls.

I have noticed that many providers will advertise in the classified section of newspapers and even some local magazines. These ads are usually much cheaper but there is a reason: They are tucked away in the back, and many readers don't bother to look through them unless they are actually looking for a particular service. I suspect most people don't look there for mental health services. Still, it can be useful. What I suggested to some colleagues who were starting divorce support groups was to share the costs, take out a double-sized ad, and promote the very specific service. In other words, I would use this inexpensive location to repeatedly advertise a specific group or workshop series. The exception is if the newspaper creates a special professional classified section, especially if it is located in a human-interest, parenting/kids, or lifestyle section of the paper where readers will see it regularly. In fact, push your paper to do this and they will probably generate more health service advertising. I like the competition — having a large number of professionals advertising significantly increases the likelihood that readers will look at the ads and be prompted to think about their needs for services. The challenge is for you to develop an effective ad that can hold up against the competition.

In addition to print media advertising, the rest of this chapter will also discuss Yellow Pages advertising, brochures, and newsletters.

DESIGNING YOUR ADS

Levinson (1990) recommends these seven steps to creating advertising that works:

1. Find the inherent drama within your offering. What makes your product or service desirable? Why would people want to buy it?
2. Translate that inherent drama into a meaningful benefit.
3. State your benefits as believably as possible. It's not just honesty, it's believability that counts.
4. Get people's attention. And make sure their interest is focused on your product or service, not the advertising itself.
5. Motivate your audience to do something. Tell them where to drive, who to call, where to write — but also tell them to make that call.
6. Be sure you are communicating clearly; 100% of your audience should understand the main point of your advertising. Zero ambiguity is your goal. (I test my ads on other local business people to make sure they get exactly the message I'm trying to convey.)
7. Measure your advertising against your creative strategy. Each promotional effort should have a simple creative plan that spells out the purpose of the advertising, the methods to be used, and the "personality" of the ads.

It is interesting to note how psychological these concepts are; as mental health professionals, you should be very good at creating effective advertising once you make a commitment to the concept.

Most texts on advertising will emphasize keeping ads simple, using a minimum of text with lots of white space to set off your main point. But I believe mental health advertising requires a different set of rules, because many people do not understand who we are, what we do, and how it can help them. Therefore, I recommend ads that are more wordy than usual, with a recognition of the need to educate the consumer while promoting your services. This is particularly challenging. One of the ways I usually deal with this is to use larger space, doubling the standard business-card-sized ad. You can provide the reader with some research-based information (e.g., the impact of divorce, marital conflict, depression; the incidence rate or the typical symptoms of your targeted problem; expected outcomes from treatment). I like to use quotes in most of my promotional material. People identify with them and feel as if you really understand their problem when they read the words they often use, which is a valid message to give. We do have a special understanding of their issues as well as skills that are proven to be helpful. Avoid using professional jargon; it's a real turn-off.

One of the most effective advertising designs is a large-print question at the top of the ad (or brochure or flyer). From the obvious "Are you looking for a good therapist?" to "Do you have an 8-year-old daughter who lacks friends?," questions inevitably pull appropriate readers to the copy of the ad because of our tendency to answer the question and then read on. It is effective for a range of issues: "Do you think your child has ADHD?" "Do you find it difficult to leave your house?" "Are you finding it harder to make decisions?" "Do you worry too much?" "Would you like to learn how to deal with food?" I'm sure you can easily add to this list. The style should be conversational, as if you were talking directly to the reader. The content of the ad then flows from the question, providing readers with some general information on the subject that helps them to confirm that you are talking about their particular concern, that you are knowledgeable about the topic, and that this is nothing to be embarrassed about. Then you describe what services you are offering and what benefits readers may get from them. Finally, you encourage them to call you.

Speaking of phone calls, many professionals find it very effective to offer free informational materials about the problem, such as articles you have written or packets offered from national organizations. This gets people to call, even if they are not looking for your services at this moment, and enables you to send them a mailing, which establishes a connection and allows you to provide them with more information about your services.

Figures 1 through 4 (pp. 98-101) contain samples of my ads, including some that have generated referrals and some that didn't, plus a couple of our group ads, which have been very effective. The key with the group (Needham Psychotherapy Associates) was coming up with the theme "Finding the right therapist takes only a single phone call." We use this in all of our promotional materials and it is becoming increasingly associated with our specific group. Having a phrase as part of your identity is a terrific goal in advertising.

In addition to reading this book and some of the resources on marketing that are listed in Appendix B (pp. 133-134), another very practical way to educate yourself on writing effective advertising is to look at print media ads and evaluate which ones you respond to. Focus on the size ads you are likely to use and identify what it is you like (or dislike) about each ad and collect notes and samples to use as a reference.

YELLOW PAGES

Yellow Pages hit the very hottest of prospects — the consumer is looking for the service. You don't need to educate as much as you need to convince the reader to select you from among the competition. But the important question is, "Just how effective is Yellow Pages advertising?" It is my experience that this varies according to your geographic area rather than your advertising skills. Some therapists report very positive results in their community; many others report very little return. Personally, I don't like Yellow Pages advertising because I can't make changes in the ad during the course of the year and it is costly in more populous areas. The best measure I'm aware of to help you decide is to ask to see copies of the ap-

CHANGING A CHILD'S BEHAVIOR

This is often the goal of parents whose child has social problems, difficulties in school, or seems sad or anxious. Meeting with me for just a few hours will result in a better understanding of the problem and produce strategies for change.

Call now: 617-444-3450
Kalman M. Heller, PhD

Needham Psychotherapy Associates • 992 Great Plain Avenue • Needham
Helping Children, Families, Couples, and Adults Since 1968

HAVING CHILDREN IS WONDERFUL . . .
BUT IT DOES PRESENT A CHALLENGE!

For help with parenting — or with the impact children have on marriage — consult with a child psychologist who has been helping for 28 years.

Kalman M. Heller, PhD
Needham Psychotherapy Associates
617-444-3450
992 Great Plain Avenue • Needham

Marital Enhancement Therapy

Did you know that marital problems are a primary cause of children's learning and behavioral problems?

A significant contributor to medical bills?
The leading cause of job dysfunction?
Or that marital therapy improves intimacy and communication and reduces conflict for most couples?

Marital Enhancement Therapy
is a time-limited (12 sessions) approach that offers the following:

- Learn about the personal "baggage" brought to the beginning of the relationship.
- Learn how gender differences can contribute to your problems.
- Clarify issues of power and control.
- Develop more effective communication and negotiation skills.

Kalman M. Heller, PhD
Clinical Psychologist
992 Great Plain Avenue • Needham
617-444-3450
Over 20 years experience in working with men, women, and children.

Figure 1: Effective Ads

PSYCHOLOGICAL TESTING

CAN ANSWER QUESTIONS ABOUT

- Learning Problems — Children & Adults
- Kindergarten & First Grade Readiness
- Children's Emotional Problems
- Marital Problems
- Career Choice & Job Problems

KALMAN M. HELLER, PHD
CLINICAL PSYCHOLOGIST
25 Years Experience
Complete Psychotherapy Services
617-444-3450
992 Great Plain Avenue
Needham, MA

If you need help
with marital problems, parenting challenges, or a child struggling academically or socially, then you want the assured competence and caring help from a psychologist with 25 years of experience.
Call 617-444-3450
and make an appointment with
KALMAN M. HELLER, PhD
Needham Psychotherapy Associates
992 Great Plain Avenue
Needham, MA 02192

KALMAN M. HELLER, PhD
Clinical Psychologist
Providing the following services since 1968:

- Evaluation of children with behavioral, emotional, or learning problems
- Individual therapy with children, adolescents, and adults
- Marital assessment and therapy

992 Great Plain Avenue, Needham 617-444-3450

Raising children can be very stressful
A psychological evaluation and new strategies at home or in school can relieve that stress.
Kalman M. Heller, PhD
Child Psychologist
Serving children & their families since 1968
617-444-3450 — Needham

Figure 2:
Ineffective Ads

NEEDHAM
PSYCHOTHERAPY
ASSOCIATES

Finding the Right Therapist Takes Only A Single Phone Call.

You want to solve a personal or family problem, but . . . will the therapist have the right skills, personality, schedule, insurance eligibility? Needham Psychotherapy Associates has **13 therapists** covering over 50 specialties across all ages, all the local and national insurance carriers, and someone available at all times for emergencies. Many therapists offer evening and weekend appointments.

You only have to call one person, **Naomi Litrownik, LICSW** at **617-449-7522**. Naomi will recommend which therapist would best meet your needs and have that therapist call you within 24 hours. The first step is often the hardest. We make it easier for you.

Needham Psychotherapy Associates

992 Great Plain Avenue Kalman M. Heller, PhD • Naomi Litrownik, LICSW • Ethan Pollak, PhD • Susan Schenberg-Templer, LICSW • Jeffrey Bradley, LICSW • Kimberly A. White, MD • Pamela Slater, PhD • Sanford Portnoy, PhD

87 Chestnut Street Joseph Rubin, PsyD • Andrea Masterman, PhD • Erlene Rosowsky, PsyD • Darlene M. Corbett, LICSW • Jody Comart, PhD

Figure 3:   Our Very Successful Group Ad

Finding the Right Therapist Takes Only A Single Phone Call.

You want to solve a personal or family problem, but . . . will the therapist have the right skills, personality, schedule, insurance eligibility? Needham Psychotherapy Associates has **13 therapists** covering over 50 specialties across all ages, and someone available at all times for emergencies. You only have to call one person, **Naomi Litrownik, LICSW** at **617-449-7522**. Naomi will recommend which therapist would best meet your needs and have that therapist call you within 24 hours. The first step is often the hardest. We make it easier for you.

Meet one of our therapists

An experienced social worker with a background in child guidance, Susan Schenberg-Templer describes herself as providing a "family practice" model. Her skills are varied in that they include play therapy with children, therapy with adolescents with a special interest in early adolescence, couples, and families.

Women's issues are highlighted in her practice including mother/daughter relationship issues of self-esteem, weight control, and history of childhood sexual abuse. Smoking cessation and compulsive shopping are among her interests in addictive behavior.

Supervision of professionals in a multi-disciplinary and multi-cultural setting lend to an appreciation for cultural diversity.

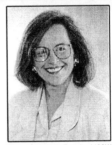

Susan Schenberg-Templer, LICSW

Needham Psychotherapy Associates

992 Great Plain Avenue • 87 Chestnut Street • NEEDHAM

Figure 4:
A Rotating Introduction to Each of Our Therapists

propriate section from the past 3 or 4 years and see how many therapists are doing repeat advertising. If there is a lot of turnover, it is a clear message that others have not found it useful and you should invest your money elsewhere.

If you decide to advertise, C. Browning and B. Browning (1986) suggest "in column" ads as the best buy. They claim people peruse the columns regardless of the stand-alone ads. Unfortunately, there are no meaningful data that I'm aware of to provide guidelines. So stick with my "repetition gauge" to assist in your decision. The only exception to this is if you live in an area where there has been very little advertising for mental health services and/or if the previous advertising is clearly of poor quality. Then you may have to give it a try. One plus is that there usually are discounts for first-time users, so the first year may not be too costly for you to see what works.

All the principles of good advertising apply here as well, but there are a few extras. Make sure your ad is at least as large as the largest equivalent mental health ad (solo vs. solo; group vs. group) and, if you're a solo practitioner, use a photograph. In personal service businesses, photographs are generally a plus. I didn't list this under print media ads, however, because it requires a lot of space, and in most newspaper and newsletter ads, you may not want to give up your informational text. You will use repetition to breed familiarity. If you do use a photo, invest in a professional photographer. Otherwise, your ad still needs a headline that grabs the reader's attention and you still need to educate, be warm, be conversational, and emphasize benefits. An article in *Psychotherapy Finances* ("Why Do Some," 1996) provides a critique of sample ads that is very helpful.

CREATING BROCHURES

Brochures should be an essential part of your promotional strategy. Whether describing a specific service, explaining who you are and what you can do for people, or presenting a group practice with its broader range of services, it is one of the most effective ways of "spreading the word." Brochures can be left in your waiting room, distributed at presentations, included in direct mailings, sent to a new patient or prospective patient, and handed to people at meetings. People like them because they combine brevity and easy handling with the extra information that they are often seeking. You as a therapist should like them because they are a relatively low-cost way to tell referral sources and prospective patients who you are and what you do.

The challenge is to use the traditional six panels effectively. I recommend that for your first brochure you work with a low-cost graphic designer (who will also know about being the operator of a small business). This will be a learning experience. After that, you can do most of your own design work, although I continue to use my graphic designer for final prepping. One of the most helpful experiences for me in working with a professional was her focus on making me define the purpose of the brochure and helping me to sharpen my message. By interviewing me about my product ("Marital Enhancement Therapy" [MET]) or the group, each brochure became a clear and effective expression of the central message regarding each topic. My goal was to communicate a sense of warmth and caring while conveying information about the way I (or we) could help solve problems. Figures 5 and 6 (pages 104-105) will show you my MET brochure.

The paper chosen is soft, speckled, and very light gray to give off a feeling of warmth and to avoid looking slick. The logo is used by the group practice; it appears on our stationery, our group brochure, and on my stationery and cards. This helps to create a visual that connects all of us and reinforces being part of a group as well as an image of caring and making things "whole." All of our brochures use the same paper, again to create a consistent image that people come to identify with us. Each brochure is two-color, with the second color different so it is easy to identify. For MET, I used burgundy for all the headings (the name and the five questions) plus my identifying data on the bottom of the front panel and the emphatic statement under the box.

I chose not to lead with a question (unlike the Needham Pschotherapy Associates brochure which reads: "When Do You Need A Therapist?") because I felt the name of the product was strong enough to draw the interested reader. The subheading immediately tells the reader two key points — this is a

Marital Enhancement Therapy

A Structured Approach to Helping Marriages Succeed

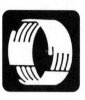

"What's a good marriage?
A safe haven where each
partner feels accepted and supported.
That's what I help couples achieve."

Kalman M. Heller, PhD
Clinical Psychologist
617–444–3450

Who Is Dr. Heller?

He is a clinical psychologist with over 25 years experience in helping children, families, and couples.

Dr. Heller is an exceptional listener and a creative problem solver. He has a special knack for translating psychological terms and theories into everyday language. And always with a sense of humor!

His column, "ParenTalk," appears in several local newspapers.

Insurance accepted.
Office hours:
Monday - Friday
8:00 a.m. - 6:00 p.m.

Telephone: 617–444–3450
Kalman M. Heller, PhD
Clinical Psychologist
992 Great Plain Avenue
Needham, MA 02192

Does This Describe Your Marriage?

" . . . We keep arguing about the same things and nothing changes."

" . . . We never talk anymore."

" . . . We haven't made love in weeks."

" . . . We never have fun anymore."

If so, then
Marital Enhancement Therapy
CAN help.

Figure 5: "Outside" Panels of MET Brochure

Can Marital Therapy Really Help?

Yes! The vast majority of people who come in have a stronger marriage at the end.

By making the initial appointment you have already taken a positive first step towards getting your marriage back on track.

For more information, call 617-444-3450.

What Happens During the Sessions?

During the first meeting you and Dr. Heller will discuss your specific marital concerns, and together, establish goals for the therapy.

The sessions cover:

- Your personal histories — examining the issues each of you brought to the relationship.

- What brought you together and why you really decided to marry.

- The evolution of the marriage with its strengths and weaknesses.

Homework assignments are given throughout the program to help increase insight and understanding.

At the end of 12 sessions you and Dr. Heller will evaluate whether further appointments are needed.

What Is Marital Enhancement Therapy?

. . . A 12-week program that helps a couple learn how to effectively communicate and resolve problems.

"Couples typically come to see me after spending years trying to change each other. I focus instead on helping them change the relationship."

Marital Enhancement Therapy helps a couple examine the values and priorities of each partner, resolve issues of power and control, and learn how gender issues impact the relationship. There is a constant focus on improving communication skills.

"It's a myth that a good marriage does not have conflict. The essence of what I do is give a couple the tools to work through conflict as a way of achieving greater intimacy."

Figure 6: "Inside" Panels of MET Brochure

"structured" approach and it helps. Positive messages are very important. The structured aspect, explained in the inside panels, is very appealing to many couples (especially resistant husbands), some of whom have had frustrating experiences in marital therapy where they just argued a lot and not much changed. The quote on the front panel shares my vision of "a good marriage" which enables us to share a common vision of what we are trying to achieve in working together to improve their relationship.

The questions at the top of the rest of the panels makes it very easy for the reader to know where the information is and what I am explaining to them. Brochures must be as clear as possible. Using questions draws the reader along. Using quotes helps readers to identify with a sense that this is about *their* marriage. The visuals gently convey the movement from being turned away to being face-to-face and help to break up the text. I did not use a photo but I definitely would if it were a generic brochure about me. If I were to redo this brochure I probably would put a photo on the panel about me. It strengthens the sense of connection.

This is the only brochure I have, although I have thought about doing one that would describe the range of products and services I offer. However, I hand this out at all presentations (along with my card and the group brochure) and, consistent with my message that specialties don't restrict your referrals, people call me for individual therapy for themselves or their children based on having a friend hand them my brochure (which they picked up in my waiting room or at a workshop). The positive feeling that the brochure apparently conveys serves as a positive statement about me as a therapist and encourages people to want to use my services. This is what a brochure is all about.

Psychotherapy Finances ("Tips for Developing," 1995) has an excellent article on designing effective brochures. Their sample is of a more professional product and costs about twice what mine did to develop (about $2,000 vs. about $1,000). C. Browning and B. Browning (1986) also discuss in detail designing a brochure. The key points stressed by everyone are:

1. Be clear in your mind about who you are trying to reach and what the primary purpose/message is going to be.
2. Identify the "feeling" impression you want to make.
3. Emphasize benefits of the service(s), not professional credentials.
4. Use conversational language, avoid jargon, make the brochure easy to read, and make the key points as clear as possible.
5. Use visuals (including a photo) to help convey your message and to strengthen the sense of personal connection.
6. The title is very important; effective ones usually pose a question, state "How to. . . ," or introduce something new. It needs to grab people's attention.
7. Quality should be reflected in the stock you use, a lack of errors, and the printing. Don't cut corners and end up with a brochure that conveys the wrong message about you and your services.

NEWSLETTERS

This is one of those items that is still on my marketing plan but hasn't been acted upon, because I have a newspaper column that achieves many of the same goals, and because the group has had too many other marketing and business priorities before this one. Newsletters can be a very effective way to promote your practice. They combine helpful information about mental health issues with a description of your services. You should be able to convey the sense of caring and competence as well as some sense of your professional style and expertise. That can be a powerful message.

The first issue to be addressed, just as with a brochure, is to identify your target audience. Is the newsletter for prospective patients, existing patients, or one or more groups of referral sources? Next, you have a rather different choice to make, because there are companies that produce generic newsletters with a space for information about your practice. (They also produce columns.) If you decide to use one of these, make sure you don't appear to be the author, for that would be unethical.

Personally, I don't like any of the packaged materials I've seen; I would encourage you to do your own. The whole point is to convey something important about you and your practice. Using somebody else's generic (and usually very dry) writing makes the wrong statement and misses out on an excellent opportunity.

If you are not a good writer, this may not be the best tactic for you. But good therapists are usually good communicators, so your potential to "talk" to your readers should be fairly high. If you are part of a group, the writing responsibilities can be shared. Rather than creating purely original articles, you can use the space to summarize interesting and relevant research you've read in a journal or book. This can be particularly effective for targeted mailings to referral sources. For physicians, summarize articles on health psychology; for attorneys, articles on forensics or the impact of divorce; for guidance counselors, educational research, or group or classroom dynamics. I'm sure you can add to this list. The main point is that sending a quarterly or even semiannual newsletter is a great opportunity to communicate to people.

One of the other reasons for the delay in our use of a newsletter has been waiting for our office to be ready to do desktop publishing. The software has become easier and cheaper (as has the hardware — use a laser printer). Doing it ourselves will be so much cheaper and makes it possible to have more than one newsletter, targeting different populations. My original vision was for a quarterly newsletter, with two issues sent to school personnel and two issues sent to physicians. These are two primary resources that we are nurturing in our community and this plan would fit with our marketing objectives. Three pages (out of a total of four pages created by simply folding an 11" x 17" sheet) would contain articles, and the back page would feature an individual therapist and a description of the group practice. The articles may, when appropriate, describe a new service we are offering or announce news about the practice. Placing copies in our waiting rooms and using them as handouts at presentations would add to the benefits, because adults/couples/parents will also find the articles interesting.

IN CONCLUSION

Levinson (1990, 1993) recommends using as many advertising tactics as possible. He states that the key issue is identifying your target audience and then figuring out how to reach that audience. Because our audience is people who may need mental health services, we face a special challenge, since they often need to be educated about when or why to seek help or how they will benefit from the services. The majority of people have very little understanding of what we do and how it helps; plus, there is still a substantial negative bias about seeing a therapist. Remember that the majority of people who need our services either do not seek services or, when they do, turn to non-mental-health professionals for that help.

Advertising is a way to raise public consciousness about the benefits of working with therapists. The more we advertise, the more people will think about the importance of good mental health services. Your goal is to use advertising to spur people into action, to make them want to call you, and to create a sense that you understand their problem and can help. All this must be accomplished in a small space and in relatively few words. Therefore, your message must be clear and focused while designed in a way that will draw readers. Remember that advertising relies on repetition for impact, so you must make a financial commitment and stick with it. This is not a quick fix to the need for referrals; rather, it is an effective part of any long-term business strategy. Even in these days of managed care, it is a great way to reach a larger audience and generate an interest in what you can do for people. I have found not only that advertising helps my practice, but that it is fun to be creative and to experience the calls coming in from my promotional efforts.

11

Case Examples

From my workshops, I have selected several examples of marketing consultation that may be applicable to your situations and provide some additional understanding about how marketing can be used to develop your practice.

CASE #1

The therapist had taken a course in pain management and developed a collaborative relationship with a chiropractic group. They made referrals, but very few patients were following through. I recommended offering free lectures on pain management for the patients of this chiropractic group as a way to introduce them to the concept. In addition, we discussed a brochure that would explain who would benefit from these services, what the benefits would be, and what the services were. Mailing the brochure with a cover letter to the patients would provide helpful information and create a connection with the therapist. The brochure should also be placed in the waiting room at the base of a small poster informing patients about the free group consultation.

There was a second issue in this particular case related to my earlier discussion about qualifications. The therapist, in my opinion, had not become sufficiently trained in the area of pain management. I recommended taking a more intensive program in this area including arranging for supervision until a higher level of expertise was reached. This addresses the issue of risk management. Entering a new area of clinical services requires special attention to these issues. Although all clinicians must be familiar with the topics of liability and risk management, I recommend reading Bennett et al. (1990).

CASE #2

The therapist had a strong background in treating the severely mentally ill, but referrals weren't coming in at a sufficient rate and it seemed like a difficult target group to market to. True, direct marketing might not be appropriate, although certainly not out of the question. Ads or brochures that might focus on particular symptoms could reach this population, or, more importantly, might reach the spouses or parents of these patients and result in referrals. The issue is that a relatively small percentage of private practitioners are interested and skilled in working with this population, so it is an area of potential. This last point led to one of my recommendations. A good source of referrals could be other therapists who have identified a severely troubled family member but don't wish to provide the therapy. I recommended developing a regular mailing to therapists in a reasonable geographic area describing the therapist's interest and expertise in treating the severely mentally ill and urging them to use him as a resource.

Because there has been a significant increase in the range of partial hospitalization programs, combined with the emphasis on short-term residential services, the therapist also needed to meet with the clinicians who were responsible for discharge planning at local facilities. An effort should be made to be part of the ancillary staff of as many facilities as possible, to attend rounds and lectures, and to offer to supervise or make presentations in order to become known. Professional publications and presentations at professional meetings are helpful if your

primary target for referrals is other mental health professionals.

CASE #3

A therapist had designed a brochure to market a product
called "Parenting Yourself," subtitled "A Structured Approach
to Psychotherapy." The front panel contained the following list
of statements: "Are you unhappy and self-critical? Does perfectionism and/or procrastination slow you down at work? Does
your anger eat you up inside . . . or cause you problems on
the outside? Do you avoid making commitments in relationships? IF SO YOU MAY NEED HELP IN" — then came the
title, subtitle, and a logo depicting an adult figure holding the
hand of a child figure. The inside panels of this first draft are
reproduced in Figure 7 (p. 114).

I noted that the brochure was much too wordy and lacked a
clear focus. I commented: "Who are you trying to reach and
what primary message do you want to get across? There's just
too much here. This is too intellectual; not warm, caring, and
helping. You need to use words or phrases that the reader can
identify with — recognize as what they have said to themselves.
Make them feel as if you know them without ever having met
them, which will elicit a feeling of trust that increases the likelihood of their calling you.

"You refer to a 'structured approach' but never explain what
that is in simple terms and how that benefits the patient.

"I think there has been an overuse of the concept of 'inner
child' in the media and it may turn people off. You need to be
clear that you are treating the adult who has come to see you.
Don't get too 'cutesy' or overuse jargon. Everything should be
written in the simplest language you can use. Most people relate to the idea that their parents' attitudes and relationship
with them is an important influence. However, they may not
realize the ways in which that might still be affecting their
lives, and that's an important point you need to emphasize in a
simple, clear manner.

"You have another key point — the one you are trying to
use as a hook — that we are too hard on ourselves, which pro-

THE PROBLEM:

A common myth is that to be an adult is to leave childhood behind. The truth is that each of us carries within our mind, a large component of childhood experience. This "inner child" is the part most connected to our emotions and provides us with energy and passion for living. Each of us also has within us a more rational "inner parent," modeled after our original outer ones. The job of our inner parent is to care for our inner child and to help guide our decisions in the world at large.

The inner parent and inner child interact within our minds in the form of conversations, most of which are subliminal. We become aware of them in times of inner conflict, such as when "part of me knows I should do this . . ." but another part of me wants to do that."

If our reason and emotion are generally in harmony, our life will feel balanced. If they are in frequent conflict, however, our life can feel out of control.

In each of these four problem areas, the inner parent and the inner child are at odds with one another. In each situation, the problem is caused by:

NEGATIVE INNER PARENTING

1. IF OUR INNER PARENT IS CRITICAL, OUR INNER CHILD WILL TEND TO FEEL UNHAPPY, ANXIOUS, AND NEVER QUITE "GOOD ENOUGH."

2. IF OUR INNER PARENT IS PERFECTIONISTIC, OUR INNER CHILD WILL TEND TO "REBEL" BY PROCRASTINATING.

3. IF OUR INNER PARENT IS ANGRY, OUR INNER CHILD WILL TEND TO BE FEARFUL — YET ANGRY UNDERNEATH. IF THE ANGER IS KEPT INSIDE, STRESS SYMPTOMS LIKE HEADACHE, HYPERTENSION, AND GASTRIC DISTURBANCES MAY RESULT. IF THE ANGER IS EXPRESSED OUTSIDE, FREQUENT TEMPER OUTBURSTS MAY OCCUR.

4. IF OUR INNER PARENT IS NEGLECTFUL, OUR INNER CHILD WILL TEND TO FEAR THE DEPENDENCY INVOLVED IN CLOSENESS AND COMMITMENT. HAVING LEARNED INDEPENDENCE EARLY, THIS INNER CHILD WILL FEAR BEING TRAPPED AND THEN ABANDONED BY ANOTHER PERSON.

THE SOLUTION:

Since negative inner parenting is the source of these problems, the solution will be found in

POSITIVE INNER PARENTING.

Traditional psychotherapy achieves this through a corrective parenting experience with a therapist. While highly effective, it often neglects to involve the client directly in the task of self-parenting. The result is that therapy often takes longer than necessary.

PARENTING YOURSELF

makes positive self-parenting a central goal from the beginning and provides structured experiences to achieve it.

INDIVIDUAL SESSIONS
utilize discussion, hypnosis, and home practice to identify negative patterns of inner parenting and develop more positive ones.

GROUP SESSIONS
are structured, supportive, and time-limited groups in which participants help one another become better self-parents. If you are currently in therapy, you are welcome to join a PARENTING YOURSELF group as a way to further enhance your progress.

Figure 7: "Inside" Panels of Draft of Brochure on "Parenting Yourself" duces feelings or behaviors that are problematic. You want people to identify with a few simple expressions of those feelings and problems, then hit them with how your new solution will lead to changes. Spell out some of the changes (remember the emphasis must be on benefits) to make people interested in choosing your services. One point you don't make that is critical: This is a short-term way of making long-term changes, that is, changing those inner tapes opens the door to enduring changes because your approach focuses on a key, underlying determinant of our self-image."

The therapist used these comments and additional feedback to produce an improved brochure, reproduced in Figures 8 and 9 (pp. 116-117). However, it was still too wordy and unclear if the concept of *Parenting Yourself* would really make a strong-enough connection to people's experience of their problems to encourage them to make the phone call. The therapist created an ad using the key concepts and the logo and gave it a reasonable trial before deciding it wasn't working. He then focused on the self-talk aspect and redid his promotional materials. In a recent conversation, he said this was working much better. This underscores one of the critical issues in developing promotional strategies. Keep working at it until it becomes effective. This therapist had a vision; it just took a few trials before he found a way to convey his message effectively.

CASE #4

A therapist with a specialty in eating disorders wanted to increase the size of her practice. This is a potentially good specialty, but it has become very competitive, and not only among therapists; many hospitals successfully promote such programs because, in more severe cases, medical treatment, even hospitalization, may be an essential part of the treatment. The advantage, as always, for the individual therapist is the ability to build relationships with potential referral sources. Also, many people prefer the more personal and private office of a therapist over going to a hospital. I recommended developing two sets of educational materials, one for physicians and school counselors (high school and college), the other for par-

Do You Talk To Yourself This Way?

- ◆ YOU'RE SO *STUPID!*
- ◆ IT'S ALL *YOUR* FAULT!
- ◆ YOU'LL *NEVER* GET IT RIGHT!
- ◆ STOP FEELING *SORRY* FOR YOURSELF!
- ◆ DON'T BE SUCH A *BABY!*
- ◆ SNAP *OUT* OF IT ALREADY!

**If You Are Saying These
Things To Yourself
You Need Help In**

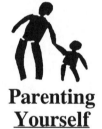

Parenting
<u>Yourself</u>

**A Short-Term Way To
Make Long-Term Changes.**

**Figure 8: New Front Panel for Brochure
on "Parenting Yourself"**

The program has two separately, yet integrated parts.

Individual Counseling

helps you to identify both the positive and negative aspects of your self-parenting style. Using a powerful combination of active discussion, guided hypnosis, and home practice experiences, you will find yourself becoming a more positive self-parent after only a few sessions.

Group Counseling

is an 8-week group program in which you and other participants help one another to become better self-parents. Each 1-1/2 hour meeting is carefully planned to provide a balance of emotional sharing and support as well as specific skill building.

If you are currently in therapy, you are welcome to join a PARENTING YOURSELF group as a way to enhance your progress.

In each of these problems, the common element is a continual, yet often subliminal, pattern of self-critical thoughts which creates physical, mental, and emotional distress.

Solving these problems requires that these negative thoughts be replaced with positive ones. Simply put, it requires that you become a more positive self-parent.

Parenting Yourself

is a short-term approach to psychotherapy which focuses on helping you become a more positive, caring parent to yourself. This unique program will open the door to enduring changes in the way you feel and behave.

Our parents often tried the best they could to guide us in life. But a child's mind is like a sponge, taking in both the positive and negative messages that parents give. The result is that each of us has an *"inner parent,"* a voice which talks to us in both positive and negative ways.

The more supportive our self-talk, the better we feel. The more critical our self-talk, the more unhappy we will be.

In fact, negative self-talk is a major part of such diverse problems as:

- ◆ STRESS
- ◆ ANXIETY
- ◆ LOW SELF-ESTEEM
- ◆ DEPRESSION
- ◆ CHRONIC ANGER
- ◆ HYPERTENSION
- ◆ SHYNESS
- ◆ LONELINESS
- ◆ OVEREATING
- ◆ ALCOHOL/DRUG USE
- ◆ PERFECTIONISM
- ◆ PROCRASTINATION

Figure 9: New Inside Panels for Brochure on "Parenting Yourself"

ents, teens, or adults. Both need to emphasize how to spot the signs of an eating disorder, but the former focuses a bit more on your credentials. Also, both need to describe your treatment program, ideally with an element that distinguishes it from other eating disorder therapies, but the one for prospective patients needs to put a greater emphasis on the benefits of treatment.

Personal selling is critical here. Regular meetings with internists, gynecologists, and high school and college counselors are the cornerstone of the marketing strategy. A helpful promotional technique would be introducing a self-administered questionnaire that these people could use to assist in identifying people with eating disorders. You provide the questionnaires, training in administration and scoring, assistance in brief intervention, and criteria for when therapy or more serious interventions are needed. If you are going to target college students, have an office near campus or on a public transportation line that students can access. For high school students, who want their autonomy, be within walking distance. (Obviously, you may need more than one location. Subletting an office of another therapist can achieve this economically.)

Many local papers have a health column. Write a piece on eating disorders and try to get it published. Lectures for concerned parents will draw good crowds, and don't forget to address the parents of preteens on prevention as well as early signs. Ads can be effective with a heading "The six signs of eating disorders."

CASE #5

This therapist was also an attorney (a surprisingly common dual career) and had extensive training in divorce mediation, which seemed like a sure winner with his background. His problem was that he didn't really enjoy mediation and wanted to shift the focus of his practice to other divorce-related services. I recommended developing a four-session psychoeducational program for teaching people how to deal with the six most difficult issues that come up during the divorce process (issues to be determined). This would be a cash-only service and could be done individually or in groups. It could be promoted in a number of ways: ads, brochures, talks, articles, and working with potential referral sources (especially attorneys and clergy) and could take advantage of his dual training.

In addition — and partly a second-tier service for people taking the psycho-ed program — I suggested organizing divorce support groups. These could be for men, women, or co-ed and should probably be time-limited but renewable for those who want to continue. It would be promoted through the same tactics and could be tied in with a child specialist who offers children's groups. Again, this is a nondiagnostic service, meaning out-of-pocket payment. The final related service could be adult therapy groups for those who need help in dealing with relationships. What is interesting here is the potential for a package of related services to be put together, creating strong promotional potential and taking advantage of this therapist's dual professions. He can build a powerful "expert" strategy.

CASE #6

This therapist had just moved into an affluent, rural community. Her specialty was group therapy. She brought in a copy of the local Yellow Pages, which clearly indicated that there were a number of established group therapists in the area. She had created a brochure "About Group Psychotherapy" and wanted to get one generic adult group started. I thought she was facing a very difficult task. Private groups are hard to get started because you need a sizable pool in order to create a compatible group, and, with no established sources, promotion would be a long process. Her brochure was rather bland and didn't differentiate her from the competition. During the consultation, I always search for anything unique about the person that can be used as a promotional edge. In this case, the therapist was a former nun. Clearly this might give her an advantage in working with the local clergy, and I recommended she begin to meet with them and ask what services they felt were needed in the community. There is especially an opportunity to integrate therapy and spirituality, which she would be uniquely suited to offer as a group experience. She might get a number of referrals from clergy if she could create a defined product with a defined outcome or purpose.

Additional discussion produced another specialized interest. She had worked with a number of women who had lost their mothers when they were children. I thought a group focusing on this population would be an excellent specialty product, but she would need to be able to state what this loss typically means in the lives of women and how a group could be beneficial. Of course, there is the potential for broadening this to loss of either parent at an early age and to have groups for men as well as women. Suddenly, we had identified a few potential strategies to help her establish a practice in a new community.

CASE #7

A group of eight therapists was seeking an array of advice ranging from questions about incorporating to generating more referrals. Their issues were common to many small groups. There was a lack of leadership and purpose. Current members were simply sharing space. Commitment to being in a group practice varied significantly, as did the size of the individual practices. They were trying to address issues of practice development and promotion before they had a common vision and a group of people with a commitment to that vision.

So it was back to the drawing board. First, the nonplayers had to be weeded out. The remaining core group then needed to develop a beginning business plan. New members needed to be brought in who fit the needs and objectives of the newly defined group. Becoming a group just for the "safety in numbers" strategy is a mistake. Would you invest your money in a start-up company that had no business plan? Then why do it for your own business?

CASE #8

A recently licensed therapist, after many years of working in the corporate world and raising a family, was seeking to establish a successful practice. She had a strong interest in couple's therapy, but a key component of that interest was helping couples with sexual problems. We decided this would be one of her specialties. The plan involved targeting gynecologists, urologists, and clergy as potential sources of referrals. Because she was a member of only one local panel, the emphasis on confidentiality fit the specialty. She decided to create a brochure identifying different sexual problems and their treatment solutions in order to educate her referral sources and then do a mailing followed by face-to-face contacts. The brochure could also be placed in waiting rooms to be discreetly picked up by potential patients. Consistent with the typical silence around these problems, a Yellow Pages ad was thought to be effective. Prospective patients might prefer not to be asking others for a referral. The ad, along with a potential workshop, could focus on the healthy statement of enhancing sexuality for couples, with the sexual disorders being mentioned but not focused on. The goal was to make it as comfortable as possible for couples to seek help for sexual problems.

A second potential specialty is an excellent example of the internal assessment process. This therapist was foreign born and had lived in a number of different countries due to her husband's career. However, she had been in the U.S. for many years and considered herself to be a successful expatriate. I thought there could be a potential here for expatriate counseling, for spouses, couples, and families, and in helping relocated executives adjust to their new location. This could be promoted to EAPs, human resource professionals, and possibly executive recruiters. It was a natural fit for her own work *and* life experience as well as her clinical interest. It could be a high-fee, no-insurance service — ideal!

CASE #9

This is the expert who has no referrals. She was the author of a couple of books on work-family issues and had expected the notoriety to simply generate business. But this was not a business plan. There was a notable absence of any clinical products that spun off her expertise. I recommended that she connect to some of the local work-family programs and become a regular speaker on the circuit. Then I suggested two products: a structured couple's therapy for dual-income couples and individual therapy for career women in conflict with relationship needs. I suggested she advertise in upscale print media (targeting a cash-only population who would be drawn to her expert image) and write for local newspapers. Her focus would be reworking a national level of success into a local level of success.

12

Some Tips on
Forming a Small Group

I stated at the beginning of this book that I thought the ideal way to practice was in a small group. In the 22+ years that I have been in full-time practice, all but one of those years have been spent as part of a group practice. Most of those years the group was formed simply to share overhead, cases, and case consultation, and to reduce isolation. These are more than enough reasons to be part of a group. However, as the marketplace has required an increasing commitment to approaching clinical practice as a successful business, the advantages of a small group have grown. There is more overhead to share in terms of an up-to-date computer system, a copier, and a fax, increased time and money for marketing, and the advantage of a part-time secretary to manage billing issues and assist in promotional activities. At the same time, there has been a significant increase in clinical expertise and related research that makes it virtually impossible to effectively treat a broad range of problems with the same level of competence as therapists whose practices are more focused.

The anxiety of dealing with managed care and the competitive marketplace is better faced by sharing the burdens and worries rather than by remaining isolated. The potential for generating exciting ideas for new products and sharing in the delivery of those services helps to keep up morale and reduce burnout. It is also much more efficient to share a case with someone on premises than to try communicating with someone at another location. Case in point: The wife of a couple I am seeing has obsessive-compulsive disorder (OCD) and I thought she would benefit from a brief intervention by a behavioral therapist in our group. With the patient's permission, I simply left the file in the therapist's mailbox for her to review. This resulted in a quick treatment plan, a phone call, and the start of the adjunct intervention that had a significant positive impact in just six sessions. This patient preferred to pay out-of-pocket for these sessions because it was perceived as easier and more effective for her than starting with a covered therapist from a different practice.

There is some added "power" in promoting yourself as part of a group. Patients appear to have more confidence in you as well as experiencing a sense of added protection; that is, a larger net, so to speak. In addition, peer review sessions (which we now call "peer consultation") are extremely helpful in case management, especially concerning cases with significant liability risks. The vitality and professional growth emanating from these weekly meetings invigorates everyone.

Creating a group needs to be a well-thought-out process. In the beginning ours was not, because we didn't really function as a true group — our structure was simply based on who-knew-whom. Only in recent years did we develop a clear vision of what the group should look like (the types of specialists we needed and the type of person we wanted). An excellent resource to assist in this process is *Building a Group Practice* (American Psychological Association Practice Directorate, 1995). It addresses the different legal structures, group dynamics issues, operational issues, financing, and governance. Although the book tends to use larger groups for its examples (with too much overhead and bureaucracy, as far as I'm concerned), the same basic issues still need to be addressed. Woody (1989) also offers some very helpful information about forming group practices.

Everyone in the group must share in a common vision of the purpose and goal of the group. Stability is critical, so you need to try to weed out anyone who doesn't have a strong commitment to a group practice and strong community ties. You need a system for how people are brought into the group and how they depart — by request, choice, or necessity. There needs to be a good fit with regard to personalities and a healthy balance of ages, specialties, professions, and gender. The current in-vogue model is the group-without-walls (GWW). Though not recommended by MCCs because of their lack of centralized management, many GWWs, according to a recent *Psychotherapy Finances* survey ("Groups-Without-Walls," 1996), are thriving. I would guess the GWW strikes a balance between the desire for autonomy and the need for affiliation. Just be sure this type of group structure really meets your long-term goals.

An attorney with significant experience in health care corporations is essential, as is an accountant (they may be in the same firm). Your state association should be able to provide some leads, and friends can be a resource just to identify good local attorneys/accountants who may know the local specialists in health care. Do some reading and consult with your state and national associations before meeting with an attorney. The more you know up front, the less it will cost, because attorneys are expensive. Our experience points toward limited liability companies (LLCs) or partnerships (LLPs) as the best option (although I think Hawaii and Vermont still don't offer this choice), especially given our desire to keep the same structure of a group of individual practices, meaning more of a partnership without the personal liability. This model is highly flexible and allows everyone to be taxed solely as individuals while providing a structure for group contracts if desired.

For the more entrepreneurially inclined, whose goal includes a significant income from capitated contracts, the fully integrated group is a must. This means that all the money flows through the group and the therapists are employees. Another alternative with similar potential is the Managed Services Organization (MSO), which is primarily an administrative structure that can operate large, dispersed groups and provide a conduit for contracts. These group practice models are not the focus of this book. For those interested in pursuing more information, I recommend a brief overview in *The Open Minds Practice Advisor* (Berman, Randers, & Mariano, 1996) and the much more detailed eight books from the American Psychological Association's Toolbox Series (APA Practice Directorate, 1995, 1996).

If you are a single-profession group, a professional corporation (PC) could work, but that will require corporate taxes (a few states do allow mixed profession PCs). Plus, I think the best groups are those in which multiple professions are represented. This creates more stimulation in approach to cases and brings psychopharmacology in-house, which makes for much more efficient case management.

Professional liability is a complex issue at the moment for groups. There can be a significant added cost, especially when physicians are part of the group. But be wary of insurance companies trying to force higher premiums without data to prove they are taking greater risk regarding vicarious liability (that you or the group will be named in a suit against a colleague). Limited liability partnerships are supposed to have some protection against your liability for acts committed by members of the corporation. In Massachusetts, the requirements for liability coverage are supposed to be determined by the Boards of Registration of the various professions, as opposed to being dictated by the insurance companies. Remember, insurance companies will always try to get you to buy more insurance than you may need. Seek advice from your attorney and professional associations.

Be keenly aware that creating a group practice is a start-up business and not to be taken lightly. It is fraught with all the potential risks of any start-up. It requires strong leadership, a clear vision, and adequate funding to cover expenses until the group practice becomes successful (typically 3 to 5 years). A review of the issues that cause many groups to fail can be found in a recent article in *Psychotherapy Finances* ("Why Do New," 1996).

Of course, if all this sounds completely antithetical to your vision of a practice, just remember that a solo practice with a good marketing plan can still be very successful, even in today's (or tomorrow's) marketplace!

Appendices

APPENDIX A

Sample Mission Statements with Some Goals and Strategies

SOLO PRACTITIONER, OFFICE IN HOME

STATEMENT OF PURPOSE

I wish to maintain a high-quality, independent practice of 20 to 25 patients per week, continue teaching part-time at the local community college, and continue to supervise trainees in the outpatient department of the local hospital. My practice will not include membership in any managed care company or insurance plan that requires more than a diagnosis for coverage. I will take advantage of the privacy of my office to emphasize confidentiality to my patients and will use my low overhead to allow greater flexibility in setting fees and in scheduling appointments. My primary services will be: treatment of mental health professionals, treatment of business executives, and treatment of panic disorders.

GOALS

1. To maintain three to four referrals per month. All following goals serve this one.
2. To increase awareness within the mental health professional community of my specialties.
3. To increase awareness within the business community of my work with executives.
4. To increase awareness of consumers, therapists, and physicians of my specialty in treating panic disorders.

STRATEGIES

For Goal #2: Write articles for state associations' publications regarding therapy for therapists; also try to participate in panels/workshops on the topic. Obtain mailing lists from state associations of the four primary mental health disciplines (or create from directories) and develop semiannual mailings on the signs of professional burnout, when treatment is needed, and the unique elements of my treatment approach, including the emphasis on confidentiality. Continue to publish articles in professional journals on this subject to enhance my identity as an expert in this area.

For Goal #3: Maintain awareness of local and national business community by reading *Wall Street Journal,* business magazines, and local business publications as well as business section of area newspaper. Submit articles on special stresses faced by executives. Speak to/Meet with human resource, employee assistance program (EAP), and out-placement professionals. Emphasize experience, success of past work (pull together some outcomes data), confidentiality, and flexibility of schedule (early morning, late evening, weekends) to attract busy executives who generally don't use company insurance. Look at integrating a computerized assessment package into the treatment program to provide more tangible feedback to executives and to formalize outcomes data collection.

For Goal #4: Work closely with physicians who frequently see panic disorders (though not always diagnosed as such) in emergency rooms or in their office. Use capacity as part-time supervisor at hospital to arrange face-to-face meetings with physicians and to present at an occasional in-service session. Create a brochure that focuses on the "signs" of panic disorder and describes the relatively short-term, highly effective treatment program I offer. Develop ad from brochure content that will appear in newspapers of local town and contiguous communities.

SOLO PRACTITIONER WITH GOAL OF 100% CASH PRACTICE

This profile is based on a true situation reported at a national conference; the success of this therapist underscores the main message of this book — if you have a clear vision and a good business plan, you can achieve success.

GOALS

1. Frequent individual meetings with all clergy in the area; selling point, besides competence in treating range of adult/couples problems, is that many troubled people approach clergy because of desire for confidentiality. Because I do not accept insurance, there are no confidentiality issues beyond legal ones. Key is putting in the time to develop and maintain relationships with clergy through face-to-face contact.
2. Frequent meetings with family practice attorneys and probation court staff to develop strong practice as guardian ad litem (GAL) doing custody evaluations.

MANAGED CARE PRACTITIONER

STATEMENT OF PURPOSE

"My goal is to develop a practice with long-term stability consisting of 25 to 30 client hours per week producing an average of $6,000 gross income per month, derived from three to six preferred provider managed care organization (MCO) contracts with companies that demonstrate their stability through large size, insurance ownership, and emphasis on value. I am willing to invest at least $100 per month and 15 hours per week in business development. As my income increases, I am willing to sacrifice up to $1,500 per month of that increase for as long as 6 months at a time in order to continuously reposition myself with MCOs so that I can reach my goals. My strategy is to develop a quality-driven practice utilizing the quality checklist. . . , my capability with sign language, and a developing market niche in somatoform pain disorder. I will aggressively market as many managed care companies as I can find until I have 10 active contracts and then I will gradually cull my contracts to those most satisfying and remunerative to work with" (Poynter, 1994, p. 144).

APPENDIX B

Marketing Resources

American Psychological Association Practice Directorate, 750 First Street, NE, Washington, DC 20002-4242. (800) 374-2721. *APA Practitioner's Toolbox Series* (1995/1996):

- *Building a Group Practice: Creating a Shared Vision for Success*
- *Contracting on a Capitated Basis: Managing Risk for Your Practice*
- *Contracting with Organization Delivery Systems: Selecting, Evaluating, and Negotiating Contracts*
- *Developing an Integrated Delivery System: Organizing a Seamless System of Care*
- *Managing Your Practice Finances: Strategies for Budgeting, Funding, and Business Planning*
- *Marketing Your Practice: Creating Opportunities for Success*
- *Models for Multidisciplinary Arrangements: A State-by-State Review of Options*

- *Organizing Your Practice Through Automation: Managing Information and Data*
- *Practicing Outside of Third-Party Reimbursement: Diversifying for Your Future*

Behavioral Healthcare Tomorrow, 6 issues/yr., $58. (201) 285-0855.

Clancy, K., & Shulman, R. (1994). *Marketing Myths That Are Killing Business.* New York: McGraw Hill.

Covey, S. (1989). *The 7 Habits of Highly Effective People.* New York: Simon & Schuster.

Davis, J. (Ed.). (1996). *Marketing for Therapists.* San Francisco: Jossey-Bass.

Directory of Experts, Authorities and Spokespersons, 2233 Wisconsin Avenue, NW, #540, Washington, DC 20007. (202) 333-4904.

Edwards, P., Edwards, S., Douglas, L., & Douglas, C. (1991). *Getting Business to Come to You.* New York: Putnam.

Employee Assistance Professionals Association, 2101 Wilson Boulevard, Suite 500, Arlington, VA 22201. (703) 522-6272.

Home Office Computing Magazine, 12 issues, $20. (800) 288-7812.

Managed Care Strategies, 12 issues, $98. (407) 624-1155.

National Health Lawyers Association, 1120 Connecticut Avenue, Suite 950, Washington, DC 20036. (202) 833-1100.

Open Minds, The Behavioral Health Industry Analyst, 12 issues, $185. Monica Oss. (717) 334-1329.

Open Minds Practice Advisor, 12 issues, $97. (717) 334-1329.

Parker, R. (1990). *Newsletters from the Desktop.* Chapel Hill, NC: Ventana Press.

Practice Management Monthly, Ira Rosofsky, Ed., 12 issues, $30. (800) 578-5013.

Psychotherapy Finances, Herbert Klein, Ed., 12 issues, $68. (407) 747-1960.

Writer's Market (annual; found in any bookstore). Cincinnati: F&W Publications

References

A look ahead: Experts describe the shape of the behavioral health practice in 1996 and beyond. (1996). *Managed Care Strategies, 4*(1), 4-6.

American Psychological Association Practice Directorate. (1995). *APA Practitioner's Toolbox Series: Building a Group Practice.* Washington, DC: American Psychological Association.

American Psychological Association Practice Directorate. (1996). *APA Practitioner's Toolbox Series: Managing Your Practice Finances.* Washington, DC: American Psychological Association.

Beigel, J., & Earle, R. (1990). *Successful Private Practice in the 1990s.* New York: Brunner/Mazel.

Bennett, B., Bryant, B., VandenBos, G., & Greenwood, A. (1990). *Professional Liability and Risk Management.* Washington, DC: American Psychological Association.

Berman, D., Randers, S., & Mariano, W. (1996). Business and legal structures to consider for provider alliances. *Open Minds Practice Advisor, 3*(4), 1.

Browning, C., & Browning, B. (1986). *Private Practice Handbook*. Los Alamitos, CA: Duncliff's International.

Browning, C., & Browning, B. (1994). *How to Partner with Managed Care*. Los Alamitos, CA: Duncliff's International.

Fee, practice, and managed care survey. (1995). *Psychotherapy Finances, 21*(1), 1-8.

Forty practice niches you'll want to know about. (1995). *Psychotherapy Finances, 21*(10), 6-7.

Future trends: Smaller networks, stronger partnerships. (1993). *Psychotherapy Finances, 19*(7), 2.

Groups-without-walls are working — for now. (1996). *Psychotherapy Finances, 22*(11), 4-5.

Kalfel, J. (1996). How do I market my practice on the Internet? *Open Minds Practice Advisor, 2*(11), 1-3.

Koman, S. (1994). *Trends in Managed Care*. Paper presented at the annual meeting of the American Psychological Association, Los Angeles, CA.

Lenson, E. (1994). *Succeeding in Private Practice*. Thousand Oaks, CA: Sage.

Levine, M. (1993). *Guerrilla P.R.* New York: HarperCollins.

Levinson, J. (1990). *Guerrilla Marketing Weapons*. New York: PLUME Penguin Books.

Levinson. J. (1993). *Guerrilla Marketing*. Boston: Houghton Mifflin.

McBride, D. (1995). Prevalence of mental disorders in the U.S. *Open Minds, 9*(9), 9.

Mental health: Does therapy help? (1995, November). *Consumer Reports*, pp. 734-739.

Niche marketing: Helping patients cope with fertility challenges; working with hearing impaired clients. (1995). *Psychotherapy Finances, 21*(12), 2-3.

Poynter, W. L. (1994). *Preferred Provider's Handbook*. New York: Brunner/Mazel.

Rust, R., Zahorik, A., & Keiningham, T. (1996). *Service Marketing*. New York: HarperCollins.

Sipkoff, M. (1995). Behavioral health treatment reduces medical costs. *Open Minds, 9*(5), 12.

Sturdivant, S. (1990). Developing a marketing plan for private practice: Basic concepts. *The Independent Practitioner, 10*(2), 27-28.

Tips for developing a terrific practice brochure. (1995). *Psychotherapy Finances, 21*(6), 7-10.

Too many therapists and not enough work: MCOs steer patients to core group practices. (1995). *Managed Care Strategies, 3*(10), 1-2.

Why do new group practices fail? (1996). *Psychotherapy Finances, 22*(6), 3-4.

Why do some yellow page ads work better than others? (1996). *Psychotherapy Finances, 22*(3), 5-7.

Woody, R. (1989). *Business Success in Mental Health Practice.* San Francisco: Jossey-Bass.

Yandrick, R., & Oss, M. (1994). Affective disorders afflict 12 million people, costing $43.7 billion annually. *Open Minds, 8*(6), 10.

Yenney, S. L. (1994). *Business Strategies for a Caring Profession.* Washington, DC: American Psychological Association.

Zuckerman, E. L. (1997). *The Paper Office* (2nd ed.). New York: Guilford.

If You Found This Book Useful . . .

You might want to know more about our other titles.

If you would like to receive our latest catalog, please return this form:

Name:_____
(Please Print)

Address:_____

Address:_____

City/State/Zip:_____
This is ❐ home ❐ office

Telephone:(_____)_____

I am a:

_____ Psychologist	_____ Mental Health Counselor
_____ Psychiatrist	_____ Marriage and Family Therapist
_____ School Psychologist	_____ Not in Mental Health Field
_____ Clinical Social Worker	_____ Other:_____

◆   ◆   ◆

Professional Resource Press
P.O. Box 15560
Sarasota, FL 34277-1560

Telephone #941-366-7913
FAX #941-366-7971
E-mail at prpress@aol.com

Add A Colleague To Our Mailing List . . .

If you would like us to send our latest catalog to one of your colleagues, please return this form.

Name:_____
(Please Print)

Address:_____

Address:_____

City/State/Zip:_____

This is ☐ home ☐ office

Telephone:(_____)_____

This person is a:

_____ Psychologist   _____ Mental Health Counselor
_____ Psychiatrist   _____ Marriage and Family Therapist
_____ School Psychologist   _____ Not in Mental Health Field
_____ Clinical Social Worker   _____ Other:_____

Name of person completing this form:_____

◆   ◆   ◆

Professional Resource Press
P.O. Box 15560
Sarasota, FL 34277-1560

Telephone #941-366-7913
FAX #941-366-7971
E-mail at prpress@aol.com

If You Found This Book Useful . . .

You might want to know more about our other titles.

If you would like to receive our latest catalog, please return this form:

Name:_____
(Please Print)

Address:_____

Address:_____

City/State/Zip:_____
This is ☐ home ☐ office

Telephone:(_____)_____

I am a:

_____ Psychologist   _____ Mental Health Counselor
_____ Psychiatrist   _____ Marriage and Family Therapist
_____ School Psychologist   _____ Not in Mental Health Field
_____ Clinical Social Worker   _____ Other:_____

◆   ◆   ◆

Professional Resource Press
P.O. Box 15560
Sarasota, FL 34277-1560

Telephone #941-366-7913
FAX #941-366-7971
E-mail at prpress@aol.com

SM/7/97

Add A Colleague To Our Mailing List . . .

If you would like us to send our latest catalog to one of your colleagues, please return this form.

Name:_____
(Please Print)

Address:_____

Address:_____

City/State/Zip:_____
This is ☐ home ☐ office

Telephone:(_____)_____

This person is a:

_____ Psychologist	_____ Mental Health Counselor
_____ Psychiatrist	_____ Marriage and Family Therapist
_____ School Psychologist	_____ Not in Mental Health Field
_____ Clinical Social Worker	_____ Other:_____

Name of person completing this form:_____

◆　　　◆　　　◆

Professional Resource Press
P.O. Box 15560
Sarasota, FL 34277-1560

Telephone #941-366-7913
FAX #941-366-7971
E-mail at prpress@aol.com